SWIMMING SOLO

SWIMMING SOLO

A DAUGHTER'S MEMOIR OF HER PARENTS, HIS PARENTS, AND ALZHEIMER'S DISEASE

SUSAN RAVA

PLATEAU BOOKS

SEWANEE, TENNESSEE

For Joanne,

For an old-time
and wonderful friend,
Susan Rava
June 2011

Plateau Books, P.O. Box 3147, Sewanee, Tennessee 37375

Swimming Solo: A Daughter's Memoir of Her Parents, His Parents, and Alzheimer's Disease

A more detailed version of the "celeries" story was published as Susan Rava, "Celeries," *The Crescent Review* 4(2): 87–92, 1986.

First Edition
ISBN-13: 978-0-9814795-0-7
Printed in the United States of America

Plateau Books and the PB colophon are trademarks of Creative Services, Inc.

Cover image: © 2010 by Martha Carter Keeble
Book design by Henry Hamman

This book is printed on acid-free paper.

In memory of George, Dorothy, Paul, and Silvia.

For Gianni, as always.

Contents

Author's Note

Almost all family names and family caregivers' names are unchanged. Certain names and identifying traits of care providers and family friends have been changed for privacy's sake. Names of all nursing institutions have also been changed.

I have recreated conversations, events, and impressions from my journal, our records, my husband's notes, and my memory. For conciseness, I have combined certain events. Any errors of fact or interpretation are solely my own.

Some family events that occurred prior to my knowledge of my Italian in-laws' family and milieu are a composite of family history, lore, and my imagination. Other events that I knew from hearsay have been woven into this work of creative nonfiction.

Susan Rava

1

Swimming to Milwaukee
1993

I suspected that my father-in-law, Paul, was failing mentally when he set out swimming straight across Lake Michigan to Milwaukee, more than sixty miles away.

One morning in July 1993, I sat alone on the porch watching the lake for signs of what the day would bring. I wondered if the horizon would be clear enough to track oil tankers with my binoculars. What would the waves, so still and almost soundless, bring in the afternoon? My eyes lighted on a swimmer in the lake straight down from our cottage. Effortless and even, the person's crawl stroke pulled through the flat surface of the water as the swimmer aimed across Lake Michigan toward Milwaukee. I recognized the stroke, then the back of the head with its balding spot and silvery gray hair, then the man's shoulders, not broad nor muscular, an old man's back still strong enough to stroke, pull, stroke, pull out into Lake Michigan. Paul, it was Paul; it had to be Paul, who loved to swim. There on a table by the front door of our cottage lay his watch, his hearing aids, and his glasses. Paul lifted his head with each breath, then stroked as he swam toward Milwaukee.

Barefoot, I raced down the steps and over the dunes to the beach. Paul's striped towel was neatly folded at the shore, his Italian sandals next to it. I began to wave my arms and shout, "Paul! Paul, turn around! You're too far away!"

But Paul had set his aids—ears, eyes, watch—on a table where they announced that he had entered a world with no outside stimuli except the cool, calm lake to bathe him, to float him with almost no resistance on that quiet summer morning. Paul didn't react to my yelling. Then, as if an inner voice had spoken, he pulled the water to turn 180 degrees and headed back to the beach. My hard-beating heart slowed; I swallowed and tried to calm myself. What would I have done if Paul had not turned back? I took a deep breath.

Paul came ashore. He shook himself like a dog. A Venetian by birth, Paul was fair-skinned, like many northern Italians, and had little body hair. He greeted me, dried himself, slid his feet into his sandals and said, "Now I'm going for a walk."

"Wait a minute, Paul. Wait. I was really worried. Nobody knew you had gone swimming. I just happened to see you from the porch."

"I enjoy a morning swim." His English was precise in spite of his Italian accent that lingered after he'd lived more than fifty years in the United States.

"Paul, we have a rule: no swimming alone. You have the same rule in your pool at home in St. Louis. It's even more important in this big lake. Please, Paul, don't swim alone. One of us will always swim with you."

"That's nice of you. I'm going for my walk now."

I watched Paul set off along the shore, his short, contained steps like those of a European unaccustomed to the miles of unpopulated beach stretching wide ahead of him. He could walk north for miles until he reached a rivulet cutting into Lake Michigan. That would stop him because the rivulet was icy cold and too deep to ford, too wide to jump. I knew that nothing else would stop Paul. My dad had spoken to me about Paul when John and I were dating: "He won't let go once he gets an idea in his head." I had translated that to mean "difficult as a person." In the freshness of my love for my husband-to-be, I had no ears for negative comments about John or his family.

At lunchtime—Paul never missed lunch or any other meal—Paul reappeared, set his glasses on his nose, hooked up his hearing aids, put on his watch, donned a flowered Hawaiian shirt, memento of a tropical trip, and joined the family. During that summer of 1993, the visits of my parents, John's parents, two of our three children, and several of their friends overlapped for a few days at our cottage on Lake Michigan.

"Well, John," I announced as we all sat down outside at a large picnic table, "your dad tried to swim to Milwaukee. I reminded him about our 'no-solo-swimming rule.'"

Everyone's eyes were on me. In the midday sun, I saw my mother-in-law Silvia's white hair aglow; the intense light smoothed the crags and wrinkles on her face. Next to her on the picnic bench sat my mother, natty in what she called "play clothes": plaid Bermuda shorts, a shirt with matching trim, and sandals that picked up the blue in her shorts.

John looked at me. I knew his eyes were twinkling behind his sun-glasses as I made this pronouncement to the family. He always kept his sunglasses on in Michigan until the sun was fully down—something about sensitivity to light. I suspected he liked the movie star image he could project with his wavy, salt-and-pepper hair, dense eyebrows, and distinguished nose. John's looks, even the mischievous ones, are Medi-terranean.

John said, "I'm glad you told him, Suze."

"House rules, Nonno," said one of our children to his grandfather.

Paul cut a tomato, spread cheese on bread. His head bent down slightly, casting a shadow on his fine features, pointed nose, and thin lips.

From the other end of the table, my father, George, pushed back and stretched his long legs. He cleared a space in front of himself. The rest of us wore shirts over swimsuits. Dad wore a once-tan sweater that hung shapelessly from his thin shoulders, a relic from college days. "Still perfectly good," he said, when I'd quizzed him about that sweater. "Your mother's added some patches and darned the holes." He'd pulled it over his head, mussing his white hair and smoothing it with the palm of his hand. He sat tall—the senior statesman overlooking three generations of his family, in-laws, friends. Beyond the cottage lay a ravine with birch, pine, and oak trees, and past the sand dunes, shone a sliver of deep blue Lake Michigan.

Around the lunch table came a chorus, "House rule: no solo swimming," followed by "Paul," "Paolo," "Nonno," as if everyone assembled had joined a song of vacation consensus.

Paul concentrated on spearing a leaf of his salad. He circled his ankle back and forth. His feet were small and light-boned, elegant in their woven sandals. He finished his bite, picked up his glass of water. He held it with a cock of his wrist. He might have been drinking Campari in a bar in Venice. Sweeping his arm around the group, he said, "I know. I know," in a mock-sheepish tone.

John watched his mother peel a peach and share slices around the table. I claimed that day's *New York Times* crossword puzzle for rest time. The young people noted that the wind had picked up.

"White caps!" our son, Will, said. "I've got my boogie board."

"My turn to do dishes," said John. On vacation in Michigan, he loved to putter in the kitchen, arranging cheeses in a special container, preparing to barbecue. After lunch, he often set off alone on what he called a hunter-gatherer expedition to find the freshest local produce. He was triumphant when he returned with picked-that-morning raspberries for dessert or apricots sold on the edge of an orchard. For vegetables, he favored a vendor who repeated, "We know you're on vacation incognito in our village, James Whitmore or Spencer Tracy. We just can't place you. All of us vendors know. You're a celebrity." I loved how much those outings pleased John.

"I'll help with dishes, John," Silvia volunteered.

John slid on the bench to sit close to his father. "I'm going into the kitchen, Papa. You understand our no-solo-swimming rule." He touched his father's arm in a gesture new to me: light, yet calming and protective.

After lunch, everyone scattered to siestas or sunbathing on the beach or riding waves. I installed myself on a rattan couch on the veranda with the puzzle, a long summer novel, and a blanket in case I got chilly. Not ten minutes into my quiet time, I heard the steady splash of a person wading into the lake, kicking up the surf. I sat upright and peered through the pines down to the lake.

Paul was alone, swimming once again toward Milwaukee. As before, Paul eventually pivoted with a splash of kicking and swam back to shore.

A year or so later, Paul was afloat in his own inner world. Doctors tested him and diagnosed probable Alzheimer's disease. No voices, no waving arms penetrated those waters. Yet, if he tuned in, he might on occasion be the polite, accommodating gentleman of long habit—only to dive back into his own private swim, aimed at a faraway shore from which no one could summon him.

That summer of Paul's solo swims was the last time we invited him to vacation with us in Pentwater, Michigan.

2

Navigation
1994–1995

Swimming Solo is the story of a family in crisis. After years of often joyful, always productive, and occasionally complicated lives, John's parents, Paul and Silvia, and my parents, George and Dorothy, succumbed, one by one, to Alzheimer's disease. This is the story of how past family bonds carried us forward as we navigated a fourteen-year voyage that began with Paul's long, solo swim in the summer of 1993. At the same time, the promise of a future symbolized by new summers with new generations along Lake Michigan buoyed us with hope during our voyage. The tale ends with my mother Dorothy's death and my return to the beach where Paul first stepped from the dry sand to begin his long, slow crawl into the waters of oblivion. I have written this chronicle as a way to comprehend these events and our families' evolution. I have also created it as a flotation device for readers who cling to a shared past yet may fear the depths of disease as they try to protect, support, and care for their own beloved parents, friends, or partners as they age.

This book began as a journal—my own lifesaver. A social worker to whom John and I had turned for counsel as we undertook parenting our own parents recommended that I use writing for calm and clarity. My journal also established a record of our parents' Alzheimer's progression. This book's year-by-year layout is one of the few vestiges of my original journal. By 2001, when I retired from university teaching, I had decided to expand my notes into a book. While I still kept a journal to track the extraordinary twists of Alzheimer's disease, I filled in context—colors, seasons, clothing, past personalities, and stories gleaned over the years. I later turned an eye on John and myself and how we functioned as partners and helpmates for our parents' declines. The story carried me back to where it began, to the beach along Lake Michigan with John, the only companion with whom I could ever imagine traveling through life.

I have chronicled Paul's, Silvia's, George's, and Dorothy's descents into the swirling, finally fatal waters of Alzheimer's disease. Throughout, I recount the glad memories, gatherings, conversations, personalities, and contributions of our four well-loved—ordinary yet remarkable— parents.

John and I live in St. Louis year-round except in July. He and I are the oldest children from two families with three children. If birth order confers any traits, John and I both have a keen sense of loyalty and responsibility with a predilection for action. Both of us, it cannot be denied, like to be in charge. We're bossy, I think our siblings would say. We became our parents' primary caregivers for several reasons.

Our parents had designated each of us as primary power-of-attorney for medical and financial decisions in their end-of-life documents. Our fathers, Paul and George, were themselves lawyers who employed fellow lawyers to draft these documents. Although there were some provisions for joint decision making among siblings, it was practical for John and me, on the ground in St. Louis where both sets of parents lived, to take the lead.

While my mother and father were cognitively able, they organized family meetings with their lawyer and bank trust officer. My brother, George, sister, Missy, and I knew our parents' desires, were familiar with their documents, and had our own copies of them. While none of us felt particularly comfortable with the legal and financial issues of estate planning, we three siblings tried to cooperate, guided by the documents we had.

John, as a lawyer, reviewed his parents' end-of-life documents, prepared by Paul and Silvia's own lawyer. The documents spelled out their wishes and how to implement them. His siblings deferred to him, yet he was meticulous in his efforts to keep his sister, Luciana, and his brother, Albert, informed about decisions he made. From both families, we had road maps with the law as organizer. Our fathers knew well the fragmentation and disputes that unclear planning could cause. In both families, there were adequate financial means for excellent, extended nursing home care. This good fortune relieved an arena of frequent dispute within families. John and I and our sisters and brothers were the beneficiaries of our parents' careful planning and saving.

Geography also put John and me at center stage during the fourteen-year period described in this book. John's sister, Luciana, lived in the Boston area. Prior to his death in 2001, John's brother, Albert, and his family lived in the Washington, D.C., area. My sister, Missy, lived in St. Louis until 2001, when she and her husband, Walt, moved to Colorado. My brother, George, lived in St. Louis for about eight months a year and spent the rest of the year at his cottage in Italy. When my siblings were in St. Louis, they were of immeasurable support and help.

Finally, family doctors and nursing home personnel asked that one family member serve as decider and communicator. My brother could not, for example, authorize the nursing home to change my mother's medications or care in my stead without a release from me. I always signed such a document when I went out of town.

After Paul's first solo swims, from 1994 to 1996, he hiccupped along. John and Silvia took him to an Alzheimer's disease specialist at Washington University Medical School, who diagnosed the probability of the disease. Paul walked in the neighborhood daily, swam in his pool, and lay on the deck, where he loved to soak up the sun in warm weather, which lasts from May through September in St. Louis. He worked steadily on an autobiographical opus, for his life—public and private, in Italy and the United States—was full of adventures. Sadly, it was too late for him to compose a cohesive story; Alzheimer's disease had already claimed his mind. Yet, he spent hours at work on his indecipherable, illegible, handwritten document, its pages lost or accidentally thrown away by Paul himself as his illness worsened. Paul's language and organizational ability had so broken down by the time he began to write his autobiography that even the factual bits and pieces of pre-World War II history no longer tracked.

Paul had been a formidable storyteller in the years when our whole family had Sunday lunch at his and Silvia's house. In particular, he loved to tell about courting Silvia in Venice in the mid-1930s. With a wry smile, he would begin by saying he would spin a story of soup and persistence. But in the telling, he invented a would-be medieval tale of romantic conquest with three identical deeds to accomplish. I loved the "celeries story" because it transported me to a stately, enchanted Venice just before World War II, a Venice from which my husband had sprung. Whenever my dad mentioned Paul's doggedness, I harked back to Paul's clever, determined pursuit of Silvia, revealed in this quiet tale of manners. And whenever

Paul launched into his story, he addressed me as representative of the American society into which he'd moved. I recognized that he wanted me to know where he had come from, what his milieu had been, and how he had maneuvered to get what he wanted—Silvia as his wife.

Over the years, Paul embellished his "celeries" soup courtship until it evoked, for us and his friends, the life he left behind when he and Silvia fled fascism to settle in the United States—he always prefaced this story by saying that they did marry before leaving Italy. Next, he set the scene by pointing out that he had been serving in the military near Venice and had, as part of his uniform, a circular cape he swung about himself in the streets of the city and wore to tea dances in salons near Saint Mark's Square. Paul also had a sword with a scabbard. The sword, I've always presumed, was for dress parade, as it never figured in his tales.

Paul would have liked Silvia to go dancing with him at Thursday afternoon galas, but she was shy and serious about her studies of history and political science at the University of Padua, 23 miles from Venice. Paul marveled at Silvia's focus and willpower. Silvia had wavy dark hair and hazel eyes that glinted yellow or green. Silvia suggested—Paul recognized this as a euphemism for demanded—that he come to her home for a midday meal.

Paul imagined, from stories he had heard about Silvia's mother's control of her four children, that it was really the mother who wished to meet Paul in her own home. Paul had long been acquainted with Silvia. When Paul was 6 years old, his mother died, and he often spent time with his cousins, one of whom was Silvia's best friend. As for Silvia's mother, she was an imposing, beautiful figure in spite of her prematurely white hair. Paul found Silvia beautiful, too. "She's beautiful even now—though just as strong-minded as her mother used to be," he sometimes volunteered.

To go for luncheon at Silvia's palazzo the first time, Paul chose street clothes—a tie, of course, and a worsted suit, his wavy hair controlled with brilliantine. Silvia's family lived in a palazzo on the Grand Canal near the Accademia. (Tourists to this day send home postcards of this palace and ask their gondoliers to pause for a moment in hopes of glimpsing a woman on the balcony or a gondola slipping through the trap door below.) While the women in Silvia's family were not given to lingering on the balcony, their butler, Guido, often glided the family's gondola out through that very trap door at siesta time, when the family rested and he was free to find his own amusements.

The first time Paul went to Silvia's home for lunch, he arrived with the bravado of a Renaissance courtier. "Now Silvia's family lived in a classic Renaissance palazzo on the Grand Canal. Classic—three stories above the ground floor with a private gondola landing and marble steps into the foyer. Ocher or rust-colored, I don't remember. With a grand living room—marble floors, high ceilings with stucco ornaments and fresco decorations on them. Her father had the first private shortwave radio in Venice in a walnut cabinet in the middle of all the antique furniture."

Around the Sunday lunch table in St. Louis, our traditional chorus was, "So tell us about your family's palazzo."

"Well, to begin, my family bought its palazzo right away when Napoleon freed the Jews from the ghetto in the early eighteen-hundreds."

"And?" we chanted.

"It's also on the Grand Canal, some blocks from Silvia's. The same style. Our palazzo was on one side of the Ca d'Oro and my uncle's palazzo on the other side. Our family owned them both. Canaletto sketched the one where my cousins still live. But that's not the story. The story is about Silvia and me."

At the first luncheon, Guido, the butler, announced lunch. Paul, Silvia, her older sister Livia, two older brothers, and their mother filed solemnly through tall double doors into the dining room, their heels noisy on the marble floor. Silvia's mother sat at the head of the table, facing out to the canal. No one sat at the other end; that place was reserved for Silvia's father, who took his dinner with the family in the evening. A reclusive man, Silvia's father was quite old and had retired from a successful insurance career. He spent his days reading in his study. Silvia and her sister were on their mother's left; Paul was seated at her right with the two brothers next to him. Each place was ready with a gold-rimmed service plate, family silver flanking it, and glasses in a row waiting for Guido to serve the wines.

Paul and Silvia had been friendly since childhood; they often saw each other in his cousins' fun-loving home. Paul was quick to explain that most Venetian Jewish families were acquainted, if not related. As young adults, Paul and Silvia would see each other regularly at private parties. Silvia was willing—perhaps had even been ordered—to return to Venice from Padua for these functions, and Paul became her constant escort. On their walks home across Venice, through the dark, narrow passageways, up stone steps, and over bridges, Silvia and Paul talked and talked as if famished for conversation.

"Why do you stay in Padua?" Paul asked. "Everyone else who studies there comes back to Venice each night."

"Independence. That's why," Silvia answered.

"But you miss some of the parties and concerts here."

"Independence, I told you. Besides, I need time to read and study. I don't want to waste it on the train."

"History and politics—what kind of subjects are those?" Paul laughed, squeezing Silvia's elbow.

"You're interested in them, aren't you? Why shouldn't I be?" Silvia pulled away from Paul. "Since you've studied Italian politics in your law school, explain why your father is so close to the Mussolini crowd."

"Now, Silvia, I want to hear about how lunch will be at your house."

"Don't change the subject, Paul. In fact, with you in the military, you're involved with the same group as your father. I don't like them or trust them. They're playing to Hitler's people. I'm afraid of the military mood right now."

"Silvia, Silvia, let's talk about us, about how it will be when I come to your parents' home." He rested his arm over her shoulder. Together the two of them filled the narrow, cobble-stoned street that led to the Strada Nuova and to the gate of Silvia's palazzo.

"Nobody talks at meals. Maybe my mother will say something or my sister—she has a big mouth and likes her own way. My brothers will be watching you."

"Ah, that one brother of yours thinks he's so handsome with his curly hair all slicked down."

"Be careful, Paul. Watch what you say." Silvia's lips were pursed, her neck taut as she stepped to the gate. "The only sounds you'll hear are Guido's feet on the floor, silverware clicking, maybe waves on the Canal. The meal will go better if my mother doesn't begin to question you." Silvia turned the wrought iron gate handle and said, "Ciao, Paul. Eat everything."

Once Silvia's family was seated for lunch, Guido appeared with the first course, a white and gold tureen of soup that he set before Silvia's mother. He took two steps backward and waited to pass each plate as it was filled. With the first ladleful, Paul noticed that in the rosy, steaming broth there were bits of green afloat. As Paul told the story, he tried to eliminate first one culprit, then another. Not round enough or bright enough for peas. Not the limp leaves of a spinach plant. Too pale to be broccoli and too small to be zucchini, no matter how they might be sliced. Cabbage was not served in such households, and green onions belonged in the south of Italy. That left celery—the one, in fact, the only vegetable Paul would not eat. At each telling, Paul changed and expanded parts of his story, but he never learned that in English the word in the singular and in the plural is always "celery." Instead, he proclaimed each time: "There were celeries in the soup."

Silvia had warned Paul that one ate everything at the table. Guido, with a white napkin over his arm to protect against spills and the heat, set a plate of tomato broth with celery before Paul. Steam rose from its surface. The celery stopped whirling, the steam lifted, and Paul saw a broth dotted evenly with bits of the pallid, ribbed vegetable. At this point, with a twinkle in his eye, Paul would say how much he loathed celeries and then digress to tell the story of his birth in a Catholic clinic run by nuns.

Born in 1911, Paul was the second child, twelve years younger than his older brother. When Paul was about 6 years old, his mother died of tuberculosis or influenza. He loved to recount his own birth because it still seemed to him a sign of his future success with women, like those in Silvia's strong-willed clan. He explained that most children of his background were born at home, but his mother, Jewish like his father, chose a clinic run by nuns because she was rather sickly and the nursing care at the clinic was renowned. Although there was no resident doctor, one could be sent for in an emergency. The sisters, it turned out, had done little midwifery but pushed up their habits' sleeves and got ready for the delivery. Paul relished describing how their white headdresses bobbed up and down and their bat-like sleeves flapped around his mother.

"Then I emerged, with the same thick wavy hair I have to this day. My hair was the first thing the nuns saw. Then my flailing arms, my chest, and my umbilical cord, which demanded their complete attention. And then, lo and behold, I was a boy. Not a one of the good sisters had ever seen a naked man! They shrieked, crossed themselves, cried for mercy, and sent the youngest flying through the streets of Venice for my father. He arrived with one of our housekeepers in tow, shooed the nuns out of the delivery room, and covered me so that I could stay there in the clinic with my mother. The nuns waited on Mother, but they never changed my diapers. Our housekeeper moved in to do that."

Paul went on to say that after his mother's death, his father, a much older man with business connections abroad, entrusted his younger son to the aunts, uncles, and cousins who lived nearby, where Paul often encountered Silvia. Yet, he had never been to Silvia's house, nor had he met her family. At home, Paul was the darling of the household retainers, eating his meals alone in the dining room because his much older brother no longer lived at home and his father was away on business trips most of the time. As Paul had always refused to eat celery, the cook never prepared it for him in any form. Paul had been indulged for so long that he could not bring himself to eat celery, not even for love.

At the initial luncheon, Silvia sat opposite her suitor. Paul did not look up at her but began to eat his soup. Venetian soup spoons were large with deep bowls. With each dip of the spoon, red, celery-filled broth flowed into the spoon's bowl. There was the possibility that with a mere tilt of the spoon next to the bowl's edge, only broth would seep in, the celery being blocked by a barrier of silver and porcelain. That was the chance that Paul took at the first family lunch: delicate sips of soup from a half-filled spoon, eyes cast down in concentration to keep the celery out. At last, only a pink film of soup was left with pieces of celery set in it like pebbles. Paul kept his eyes lowered and laid his spoon on the service plate. Guido swept to his side immediately, taking plate and dish away. Paul looked up and out the doors to the canal and remarked on the splendid day. No one responded.

Paul understood that their silence was one of the formal customs of the household; Silvia had warned him that they did not talk much during meals. He also understood that Silvia's mother was watching him carefully.

—∞—

Silvia and Paul didn't talk about the lunch or the soup. Silvia sent Paul a note from Padua, saying that her mother hoped he would come for lunch again. Paul scrawled a reply to Silvia rather than to her mother, "Yes, with pleasure," on a gilt-bordered officers' card.

For the second time, Paul came to Silvia's house, and Guido announced that lunch was served. The family, no more talkative than before, filed into the dining room, seated themselves in the same arrangement, with Paul to the right of Silvia's mother. When she raised the top of the tureen, Paul saw red soup and, through the steam, strings from pieces of celery. It occurred to him that it was odd to offer the same first course and that Silvia's mother somehow may have learned about his preferences and was testing him. Paul sipped the broth calmly, pushing the celeries to the middle of the bowl, deciding he would leave the spoon in the dish to hide the offenders this time. Again, there was little conversation—sounds of spoons softly touching china, a chair scraping the floor, a comment on the midday breeze—nothing more. As he finished, he slid the spoon across the bottom of the plate, pushing the celery to one side with the spoon covering it.

At the third luncheon, Paul's final test—for by now, Paul had realized that Silvia's mother was taunting him—Guido held wide the double doors to the dining room as the four children, their mother, and Paul entered. Their places were the same, the shutters open to the canal, the silver shining, the tureen closed. Before Silvia's mother served the soup, he knew it would be the same. This time, his tactic was to leave the celeries in a ring around the edge; he hoped they'd settle that way as he dipped out the broth. He held his head up as he ate and watched no one, except he tried to catch Silvia's eye. She turned toward the window that gave onto the Grand Canal. Once again, Paul finished the broth without eating one bit of the wretched vegetable.

Silvia's mother laid her spoon on her service plate and rang the silver bell that signaled Guido to clear. He returned from the kitchen with a platter of veal slices laid out like fallen dominoes. Parsley bushed around the edge, and silver utensils formed an X across the meat. A garnish of vegetables followed, then salad. Paul had used all but one fork and a pearl-handled knife. Guido removed the red wine glasses and served white wine, which meant that there would be fruit, maybe cheese, then lunch would be over. The fruit came piled high with grapes, plums, pears, and colored Jordan almonds scattered at random. Grape scissors poked out from the mound. Paul feared he would send the fruit rolling across the table when he served himself.

"Let me start," Livia, Silvia's sister, said, "Paul might be afraid of upsetting things."

Silvia's mother recommended the grapes, which Guido had brought from his village the previous weekend. With the tip of her knife, Silvia flicked the seed from a plum. As it hit the plate, Paul caught her eye. She smiled and bit into her fruit.

Soon after, Paul called at the palace at teatime and asked for Silvia's hand in marriage.

Whenever Paul recounted the celeries tale, I paid rapt attention, as I had already decided I should preserve it as family lore. Silvia often clucked at the memory of herself as a young woman pursued and at Paul's delightful capacity to embellish. Occasionally over the years, John and I successfully sneaked a little celery past Paul in soups, pasta sauce, and stew.

—m—

John was not blind to the signs of his father's Alzheimer's disease. He and I both recognized that Paul could no longer spin a yarn like the celeries story. He acknowledged his father's serious memory loss when, in 1994, Paul forgot his hearing aids on a trip to Madrid. He phoned to ask John to send them via courier. John immediately dispatched the aids to his father. We both laughed and joked—naively we now realize—about the utter outlandishness of his dad's demand. When Paul summoned John to help him with taxes and insurance, John concluded that he should remove financial affairs from Paul's purview, so befuddled was his father.

As this book begins, in mid-1996, Paul had become irascible and demanding. His walks turned into aimless wandering. He told no more tales about his family or Venice. Paul was beyond forgetful; he spoke little, often so softly that I could neither hear nor understand him.

Silvia slowed down and stayed close to home. Paul grew paranoid whenever Silvia left the house. He called me several times to ask if I would telephone the police to locate Silvia when she'd merely gone out to run errands. After a few of these incidents, instead of leaving the house alone, Silvia puttered in the garden within earshot of Paul, who demanded that she type his scribbled manuscript. As the months passed, Paul's demands led to verbal explosions that Silvia tried to prevent by acquiescing to his requests. All this came to a head in mid-1996.

3

Octogenarians Are the Problem
1996

John's parents, Paul and Silvia—both in their late twenties—had arrived in St. Louis in 1940. Just as Paul and Silvia delighted in their adopted city, St. Louisans were entranced by the pair of sophisticated Italian immigrants. Paul was a dashing young law professor who had taught in Padua, and Silvia was an educated woman from a worldly background. They had left Italy on the heels of the fascist laws that prohibited Jews from teaching in the university system. Paul went first by train to England, where he had hoped to begin a business. Silvia with John and Luciana followed a few months later, as members of both of their families began to hide in the countryside, flee Italy, or convert to Catholicism. After a year in London and Oxford, where John went to nursery school, Paul received a scholarship to retrain at the Washington University School of Law. This project would take two years as he learned the American legal system. The family sailed from England for Ellis Island just before the Germans blew up several other ocean liners. To this day, I find it remarkable that a young couple with two toddlers mustered the resilience and courage to uproot themselves for a new continent and an unknown future. Silvia, for example, had studied English at the Marco Polo High School in Venice but had never contemplated spending her adult life in an English-speaking country.

As Silvia and Paul were settling into their first St. Louis apartment, a neighbor kindly suggested they put up window shades for privacy. Silvia had never heard of shades. Massive, wooden, outside shutters had closed the tall windows across the front of the family palazzo on the Grand Canal. With all the adjustments to a new culture, the Italian language continued to enfold the family like a blanket. John spoke Italian at home until he learned English at school. Then, like countless immigrants before and since, he refused to speak the Old World tongue with his parents. Italian remained Paul and Silvia's first language, the language of home. In public, Paul and Silvia's accents transformed their accustomed politeness into charming manners.

In her middle and senior years, Silvia's hair, which had turned white early, was chic: short and combed back on the sides with bangs across her forehead. She favored elegantly tailored, jewel-colored silk dresses—emerald or violet—purchased on her frequent trips to Italy to visit relatives. Her eyes dancing, Silvia loved to talk about her homeland, the United Nations and world affairs, and her children. She was a practical, can-do person. With nimble hands and a sturdy build, she could repair anything with duct tape, knit a sweater in a few days, mix and pour concrete, and lay flagstones. Before I knew her, she appears in photos as trim and fashionable. As I knew Silvia, she wore classically tailored suits or dresses for outings to the symphony or dinner parties. Yet, she was unfussy in her grooming—no manicures or weekly beauty shop appointments. She wore simple jewelry, such as a strand or two of pearls.

In contrast with Silvia, Paul wasn't handy at all, but he was equally elegant. He stood six feet tall at his prime, a slender man with light hair and blue eyes. Paul kept a comb in his pocket to tame his hair; when it turned silver gray, it stood up like electric waves, giving him the air of an intense scientist. A handsome, European-looking gentleman, Paul was tan and fit from swimming and walking.

Paul had a romantic, sentimental streak. While Silvia disdained religious belief and could not fathom faith as anything but weakness or folly, Paul treasured the Jewish legacy of his Venetian ancestors without practicing his religion. He was an activist in Italo-American affairs and Democratic politics. Throughout the 1970s, Paul served as one of the attorneys for the St. Louis Board of Education in a landmark school desegregation case, a cause he strongly supported. Whenever Paul was involved in representing a cause he believed in, he was like a dog worrying a bone—tenacious, relentless, and totally focused on winning. While Paul could be charming as he engaged in give-and-take conversation, I once heard him be short and dismissive with a friend whose opinion must have seemed ill formed. I knew I didn't want to cross him.

Paul's mercurial temperament had brought complaints from one of his law partners in the 1970s. John confronted him at that time.

Having rehearsed with me at home, John began, probably in Italian, the language the two often used together: "Papa, your law partner Hugh came to talk to me."

"Hugh? Why?"

"He asked me to talk to you about your law practice."

"About my work? About the office?" Paul was surely speaking at a rapid-fire pace by then. "Why about me?"

"Because of your behavior. The way you act."

"What's wrong with how I act? I am the way I have always been.

Nobody can say anything bad about me."

"Papa, you're talking too fast and too loud right now. That's part of the problem. You just don't stop. . . ."

"I don't know what you mean." Paul cut John off. "I've always acted the same way. I won't have Hugh or you or anyone else damaging my reputation."

"But, Papa. . . ."

"Don't stop me. When I want to talk, I'm going to talk."

"Well, Papa, if you don't slow down and cool down, Hugh says the partners in the law firm will have to take action."

"Action? Action? Who are you to talk to me about my law firm?" At this point, Paul slammed his hand on the armchair, John reported to me later.

"You will be asked to leave the law firm."

"Asked to leave? After all these years? For what? For what I've always been? For everything I've done? After everything I've done for Hugh and all of them and St. Louis? Leave? No."

"This is exactly what they mean. Right now, you are too insistent; your voice is too loud. Hugh says that you don't listen. Other lawyers in your firm and around the city are complaining."

"About me?"

"Yes, you have to get psychological help, Papa. Now. Something is not right. I've talked to Dr. Stern and made an appointment for you." John later said he spoke as firmly with Paul as when he'd practiced with me.

John told me that his father suddenly appeared deflated, as his whole body slumped back into the armchair. Tears filled his eyes. And John's too. They were both quiet for a moment.

"After all I've done here in St. Louis," Paul murmured.

"There is good medical help available for you, Papa." John had already visited a doctor to learn about the mood swings that character-ized so much of Paul's behavior and personality as we knew it: explosive, intently focused, brilliant yet blind and deaf to others, overactive then lethargic, persistent, courtly, visionary, impatient, aloof, sadly silent, then welcoming.

"I will do whatever needs to be done," Paul said.

As soon as Paul began to take medication, which he took for the rest of his life, for what was diagnosed as bipolar disorder, he was calmer and easy to be around—until Alzheimer's disease set in.

Silvia and Paul's marriage was complex: stimulating and challenging, devoted and pleasant, especially in their senior years when they enjoyed a compatible modus vivendi. The two always cut a figure around town. Together they sparkled as hosts of frequent dinner parties, their guests university intellectuals, foreign visitors, and artists. Silvia blossomed within her household as a talented cook and hostess. Guests remembered cocktails outside by the swimming pool and buffet suppers with veal scallopini and grilled peaches stuffed with sweet almond paste. People adored Silvia's cooking, her bright eyes, her alert and informed spirit. They often preferred her to the mercurial Paul, who kept his distance in spite of his Old World charm. Out of shyness and hesitation about her English, Silvia didn't develop as many activities or connections outside the home as Paul did, though she joined a few organizations and would occasionally meet a friend for lunch.

As Alzheimer's set in, Paul still remembered how to swim—almost an instinct from childhood summers on the Venetian beach at the Lido. When May came every year, he helped Silvia sweep the pool deck as they waited for the teardrop-shaped pool to fill. Then came a call to our house, just a block away. "The pool's open," Silvia announced. "Will you come this afternoon?" I loved swimming at Paul and Silvia's, especially on June afternoons when I stretched my muscles from a year of teaching to get into shape for July swims in Lake Michigan.

—⁂—

On a June morning in 1996, I lugged my in-laws' vacuum cleaner to the front door of their large, yellow brick house. My sweeper was on the fritz, spewing our basset hound's hair back onto our floors. I had borrowed my in-laws' ancient sweeper with its long handle and dangling cord; it was awkward to haul up the steps, along the walk past rhododendron and azalea bushes.

Before I could set the sweeper down to knock, the front door swung open. Silvia, 84 years old, flapped her arms and shouted, "Paul has just fallen. Hurry, hurry. Paul has fallen."

I stepped into the dining room, where Paul was draped forward on the table, his head cradled in his arms. Pat, their housekeeper, bent over Paul. Her shiny brown hands held a wet compress to his forehead. In her fifties, Pat was at the peak of her strength. She stood a solid five feet nine, carrying herself as straight as if she were in charge of all the space and events around her. If, Pat, a black woman, had been born a generation later, she would surely have pursued a career as a businesswoman or a politician. When she spoke, she was commanding. Now she enfolded Paul as she pressed the gauze against his forehead. I could see that blood had begun to seep through the compress.

Pat gave Paul instructions: "Now Paul, look up at me so I can see the cut."

Paul didn't move.

"Where—just show me where your glasses went," Pat said. Paul didn't answer. I felt myself become tense and extra alert. I couldn't tell what condition Paul was in; he looked limp, as he sprawled on the dining room table in the midst of scattered papers.

"You need to lift your head to show Susan that cut," Pat repeated gently.

Paul spoke first, "So Susan's here," and then lifted his head. I could see his shoulders relax. Paul trusted and liked me, even though I knew he would have preferred a Jewish daughter-in-law. He sat up, ready to work again. "Where are my papers?"

Silvia busied herself collecting his papers. Practical and accommodating, she restacked them with her still nimble hands. The wrinkles above her bushy eyebrows had deepened. She stopped tidying long enough to focus on Paul's forehead, where blood had coagulated over his left eyebrow. She retrieved his glasses from the floor.

"It is not serious, Paul," my mother-in-law pronounced in careful English. When alone, she and Paul spoke Italian together, but they both used English in Pat's and my presence.

"It is serious. I want my papers in the right order," Paul answered.

Pat intervened, "What would make Paul fall? You ought to call the doctor."

"Please, somebody, explain to me how Paul fell," I said, relieved that he was refocused on his work.

"He stood up from his writing and fell. He must have hit the edge of the table on the way down," Pat said. "I picked him up."

"Take this bandage off my head," Paul reached for his forehead, as he pursed his lips. "I need to get back to work."

"We must check with the doctor," Pat repeated.

My mother-in-law said, "He has never fallen before. The cut is nothing. Why call the doctor?"

"Exactly because he has never fallen before. You ought to call," I said.

"No," my mother-in-law insisted. "Paul needs to work, and we need to clear space here for lunch."

I parked the vacuum cleaner in the hall closet and ducked into the kitchen to confer with Pat. "You're right, they ought to call the doctor," I told her.

"They're going to drive me crazy," Pat said. "All Paul does is write that book of his. He makes your mother-in-law type it, then yells at her because she can't read his scribbling and doesn't type fast enough. They need a doctor."

"I know, I know. Hang in, Pat. We really need you."

I left them to pull lunch together and sort out whether to call the doctor. Little did I know that this would be the beginning of an alliance between Pat and me, a caregiving pact that often meant circumventing or overriding my in-laws' desires and efforts to preserve life as they'd known it. During the summer and fall of 1996, Paul grew sicker and sicker with what was diagnosed as Alzheimer's disease.

Instead of fretting, I tried to be breezy about the signs of aging that Paul and Silvia were showing. We were lucky because Pat, who had long experience with old people, coped well with Paul; he liked and respected her. Pat arrived at their house every morning, Monday through Saturday, and left in the late afternoon. Silvia felt easy about leaving Paul at home with Pat to go on a garden shopping trip, attend a League of Women Voters meeting, or have lunch with a friend. Thanks to Pat, Paul and Silvia's house looked tidy and clean. Paul, however, often lost his keys or stormed over his writing, exaggerated behaviors that turned out to be symptoms of Alzheimer's disease.

In fact, Paul's cut was not bad. But I asked myself why he had fallen. I wondered whether he had suffered a head rush or blacked out. I was concerned about him because he had the best balance of all four of our very old parents. In the summer of 1996, John's parents, Paul and Silvia, were both 84 years old. My mother, Dorothy, was also 84, and my father, George, was 87.

That June, those four old people, our parents, had numerous "crises." Sometimes their reports of lost keys, lockouts, and myriad ailments seemed annoying. Yet other times I rolled with them, as if I'd always been a caregiver to our parents. On occasion, however, I felt anxious as I considered whether I was equipped to deal with an increase in daughterly responsibilities, especially with my full-time teaching job.

My anxiety deepened when, only a week or so after Paul fell and cut his head, my dad telephoned. He was worried about Mom, who was suffering with shingles, a severe and painful viral nerve infection in the herpes family.

"Chickadee, Chickadee (Dad saying my pet name twice presaged serious business), your mother's not waking up." My dignified, reasonable father, who was still proud of his eye-catching, slender height and his shock of white hair, sounded like a scared child.

"What does that mean, Dad?" I answered. I tried not to reflect his panic.

"Well, the doctor gave your mother some pain medicine. Codeine or something. And she doesn't wake up."

"Dad, is she breathing and stirring in her sleep?" I said, feeling impatient.

"Yes, she is. Of course. What do you expect?"

"I expect that you just have to wait for the medicine to wear off," I said.

"Do you think shingles could be fatal, Chickadee? That they are killing your mother right now?" He sounded breathless.

"Dad, I don't think so. She's sleeping normally, you say. She'll wake up. Besides, I've had shingles, and I'm still here." I must have sounded sarcastic; I felt that way.

Damn, I chastised myself; I should have soothed his fright and reassured him that Mom had not abandoned him. Instead of being uneasy about my mom, I was flabbergasted by my dad's terror. I was used to him being confident, in-charge.

It was summertime. I set my mind on walling off my parents' crises as I went about my business. I was scheduled for an annual physical checkup an hour after Dad's call. On the way to the doctor, I gave myself a pep talk: "It's June. Your dad and mom are okay. Even your mom's shingles are better. Focus on yourself. Paul's cut is healing—put that worry aside, Susan. Concentrate on whatever's on your own mind with your doctor." Yet, for the first time in my life, my blood pressure was high. My doctor ordered me to restrict salt and monitor my pressure at a machine in the supermarket. A week later it registered an acceptable 128/78. Salt was not the problem. Octogenarian parents were the problem.

Certainly, neither John nor I ever imagined what we came to know about being point people for our aging parents.

—⁓—

As young adults, John and I had separately tried life in New York City. During law school, John had a summer legal clerkship there, but the anti-Semitism he observed made him wary of seeking a career in that city. A familiar St. Louis, which already had Jewish partners in major law firms, seemed more promising. After college, I worked with a foreign high school exchange program in New York, shepherding international students and traveling to Europe, South America, and California. However, the break-up with my East Coast college sweetheart soured me on the job and the city. The lure of a new boyfriend in St. Louis—not John—

pulled me home, but that relationship didn't work out. After living in St. Louis for two months, I met John at a political meeting where my father was the featured speaker. Dad had convinced me to go along with the guarantee of meeting interesting, eligible young men. I suspect he was anxious for me to get married because I was 24, too old to be single in St. Louis in the early 1960s.

John turned out to be liberal, cosmopolitan, energetic, and Italian-looking with his curly dark hair and heavy eyebrows. His strong opinions and sense of fun about settling in St. Louis were infectious. He invited me on dates that felt like adventures. "How about going to a chamber music concert on Monday night?" I had never been to Sheldon Hall with its resonant wood paneling. I loved the academic-intellectual combination of John in a three-piece tweed suit and the baroque music. "Want to go on a picnic in Babler Park?" I hadn't been there since I was a kid. "Will you go campaigning with me door-to-door? My buddy Chuck is running for Council." Sure, why not? My dad had been active in politics. I was intrigued enough by this man to knock on doors, stuff envelopes, and turn down admission to graduate school far away from St. Louis. When John and I began to date, a mutual friend told me that John was like an untamed colt. I found that not a warning but an attraction.

In contrast with his high spirits, I was calm and even-tempered. At five feet nine, I was only a little shorter than he, trim from my love of the outdoors, playing tennis, and swimming. I was blue-eyed and fair-haired with unruly waves not easily controlled, in spite of back-combing and rolling my hair on big rollers to try to achieve the smooth look of the day. My features were classic; John's looks were rugged and asymmetrical. John was eligible, and so was I.

I don't know whether my father knew John would attend his political meeting. I did know that my father and Paul were friends, that the two

couples were in a discussion group together. Paul and my father had been
in the same law firm in the 1940s and continued to lunch at a lawyers' table
in a downtown club. Some years before meeting John, I'd heard my parents
tsk-tsk about Paul's son, who stubbornly insisted on a year in Italy before
law school. Secretly, I'd liked the sound of that fellow. At that time, I had
been trying to convince my parents to let me study in France for a year.
Subsequently, Dad had touted John's diplomas to me—undergraduate
and law school with a master's degree in international studies, which
had provided an excuse for him to spend a year in Bologna and one in
Washington, D.C., before law school.

While John and I were having so much fun together, we soon realized
we were in love, and so we married. Our wedding was elegant and well
planned. My mom managed all the details with aplomb, and John and I
and our families and friends had a terrific time celebrating the day.

Once we were married, John established himself in his law practice,
and we had three children in the space of three years. First came Ellen,
then Will, and finally Carol. I went on to graduate school for a doctorate
in French literature and a teaching job at Washington University in St.
Louis. Our children grew up in almost the same neighborhood where
John and I had grown up, one block from Paul and Silvia's house. We dug
our roots deeply into the city. We were interwoven with family and old
friends from childhood and high school, yet John and I made new friends,
blending our groups of acquaintances. While our parents shared a love of
the symphony, theater, and politics, John and I enjoyed art galleries and
sculpture, university colleagues, a cabin on an Ozark river, and gourmet
dinners prepared with friends.

Our caregiving role was an accident of geography—neither contemplated nor expected.

One evening in that June of 1996, when John and I had been married thirty-one years, he charged into the kitchen, furious. "Do you know, Suze, that my mom spent all day hunting for my dad's khaki pants, which had his wallet in one pocket and his house keys attached to a belt loop?"

"Poor woman." I thought of Silvia on a day perfect for gardening. "How could a person lose his pants?"

"He hid them." John shook his head. "Then, on top of that, he decided to make copies of his damn book. He ordered my mom to drive him to the copy center."

I pictured three o'clock on a summer afternoon: Paul without his pants, his wallet, his keys, demanding copies of his scribbled manuscript or autobiography, which Silvia had attempted to type. Silvia probably hadn't had a moment to weed around her basil plants or read the world news in the *New York Times*.

John went on with the litany of his father's doings, then stopped: "You and I are going on our trip to France. And then to Michigan. We can't be slaves to my parents." His shoulders slumped as if defying his own resolve.

"We can't be. We can't let ourselves be. Even if your dad loses his pants."

"Not funny. Did you notice how my brother and sister were silent when I suggested they come here to help out while we're away?" John said.

"I noticed," I answered.

"Now Mom's all worked up about their trip to Italy. It's not until September. She's scared of what the relatives will think of Dad. She's worried Dad will hide stuff like his passport and shout at her or wander away."

"Oh, he will. He will do it all," I answered. "Your mother's afraid of your dad, isn't she?"

"Really afraid. I should have kept my mouth shut." John sounded sad. "But I told her not to let Papa boss her around. Then she stormed at me: 'You don't have to live with your father twenty-four hours a day. You cannot possibly understand it.'"

Physically, Paul was strong and lean from walks in the neighborhood and swims in the pool. But losing keys and hiding his pants had given way to striking memory lapses, reasoning failures, and frequent emotional outbursts. Paul, Silvia, and John had consulted a Washington University neurologist with an Alzheimer's specialty. Paul was perceptive enough to say to that doctor in 1996 that he was only "50 percent of my old self."

Already, by the mid-1990s, we understood that there were no reliable tests to diagnose Alzheimer's disease except for a brain autopsy. Doctors did, however, evaluate Paul for other treatable causes of dementia, including abnormalities of the brain, such as a brain tumor or metabolic indicators of cognitive decline. Thus, doctors narrowed the range of causes for Paul's paranoia and fears; for his aphasia (loss of the ability to use or understand language); and for the progressive decline of his intellectual abilities—all symptoms typical of Alzheimer's patients in the early or mild stage of the illness.

Tests of cognitive impairment can be done in a doctor's office; however, for a more accurate diagnosis, family members and caregivers are asked to report personality and emotional changes as objectively as possible. And so Paul's visits to physicians included three observers: John, Silvia, and Pat. Pat quickly became John's ally. While Pat and John were keen observers, Silvia tried to cover for Paul. She intervened to answer questions addressed to him and corrected his replies, so that his mental deterioration was not always evident, especially to doctors and family members who didn't see him regularly.

When John asked Silvia about Paul's behavior, she minimized his unreasonable demands, often related to his "book," and did not tell John about Paul's violent, even frightening, outbursts that, in fact, affected her everyday life. Pat reported these behaviors to John and to the doctors. While Paul had always been "temperamental," he now became unpredictably moody. In his own self-analysis, he seemed lucid and poignant as he assessed himself at "50 percent of his old self." Yet he grew less capable of elementary memory or cognitive tasks, such as counting backward, recalling a list of words just spoken, and remembering the day of the week or the date of his own birthday.

In conversations with the neurologist, Pat and John also served as Paul's advocates, which Silvia, defensive and upset, could no longer do. John understood that just as important as Paul's storytelling had been to his self-image, his "book" was equally important, no matter what his efforts produced. John reminded the doctor about Paul at the peak of his intellectual powers. As Paul's advocates, John and Pat wrote down the neurologist's analysis and instructions to review later with Silvia, whose hearing was literally and figuratively faulty. Because he was of a younger generation and less engaged in his parents' daily affairs, John brought clarity and empathy for his father's plight, his decreasing "mental percentage."

In the early fall of 1996, while John was out of town, Silvia phoned me to say that Paul had left the house, angry with her. Initially, I was resentful and mad at the possibility of missing a dinner engagement and having to deal with Paul and Silvia's problems. I hadn't yet accepted the shared roles John and I would come to play in all four parents' declines. I clung to my own activities. Yet, neither Silvia nor I had any idea where Paul might go or whether he would get lost. I took a deep breath, tried to calm Silvia, and gambled that Paul would return on his own before dark. I counseled Silvia to stay at home and call me if he weren't back quite soon. I went off to my dinner. After about forty-five minutes, she called to report that he'd returned home without explanation.

A week later, Paul wandered off with a wheelbarrow and tools to rake leaves—uninvited—in a neighbor's yard. And so began the autumn of Paul's wandering and neighbors' calls to alert us.

Silvia continued to accommodate and "serve" Paul, as she tried to maintain tranquility and prevent him from leaving the house. She drove him to the library, the copy center, and doctors' appointments. During traditional Sunday lunches at our house, Paul was nearly mute. He used his hands to show the shape of a noun he couldn't recall. He mumbled, yet we could not understand what he said.

One Sunday, I said, "Paul, I understand you visited with your old friend Gordon the other day."

Paul lifted his head from his soup, smiled at me, and descended into the mechanical spoon-sip-spoon-sip of eating minestrone.

Silvia said, "Oh, Paul was so happy at the party. He loved chatting with Gordon."

For John and me, the pleasure we had taken in his parents' company for so many years turned to a heavy autumn sadness, as they clung to what their life had once been. Paul was on a swift descent.

At eight-thirty on a Saturday morning in early December, John and I were drinking coffee, reading the paper, and listening to the news. Silvia phoned John. His half of the conversation sounded like this (in my translation from the Italian he used with his parents): "Mamma, where did Papa go?" John's anxious words rushed out.

"Out—but where, Mamma?"

I was wrapped in a heavy bathrobe in our kitchen on that cold day. John was bundled in his wool robe.

"Because he didn't cook his eggs right? What does that mean? Since when does Papa cook his own eggs?"

"Who called you, Mamma? Where is Papa?"

"Mamma, do you hear me? Do you have your hearing aid on? You can't let him just leave. Stop him. Stand up to him!"

John began to yell. He set his coffee mug down, straightened up on the kitchen stool.

"I'll get in the car and go look for him, Mamma. You stay there in case he comes home. Calm down!" John shouted.

He put a parka on over his robe, muttered under his breath in English as he gathered his keys and wallet: "My dad's a horse's ass. He can't treat my mother this way. I don't give a shit about his eggs. My mom has to stand up to him."

John slammed the door of our house and of his car as he went to search for Paul in our neighborhood that frosty December morning.

Robe tight around me, I waited in the kitchen and wondered why Silvia feared Paul so. Silvia had often commented over the years on how shy she was, how much she loathed conflict. Now, Paul frightened Silvia, or, rather, the menace of his misbehaving—verbal insults or even shoves— hung in the air as Paul's judgment waned. Over the years, I knew Paul as tenacious, yet prone to silent depression that rendered him passive. He was devoted to Silvia and dependent on her, especially in his last decade. He may have spoken too loudly as he delivered opinions on subjects about which he felt deeply, but he had always treated Silvia with respect. His Alzheimer's disease-induced behavior went beyond anything Silvia or John or I had experienced before.

I refilled my coffee. Forty minutes had passed since Silvia's call. Why, I wondered again, had Silvia never stood up to Paul? But I told myself that a woman tentative about her ability to speak English, new to motherhood, teaching herself how to cook, thrust into an unknown culture in the American heartland, whose husband needed to retool to earn a living quickly—such a woman, so far away from her family, could only stay steady and go along with whatever happened. She had adapted in her own way.

John slammed the door as he came in.

"My dad just arrived home, as if nothing had happened."

"Where had he gone?" I asked.

"Who knows? Not a clue. He headed right back to work on that so-called book."

"And your mom is frantic."

"And desperate. And furious."

So were we.

When Paul and Silvia arrived for Sunday lunch the next day, I was reminded of all the Sundays when our family—Ellen, Will, and Carol as youngsters—went up the street to Paul and Silvia's house. The vision of an Italian family gathered around the table for Sunday lunch had been part of the magic that attracted me to John. Silvia always prepared a big meal with Paul's required pasta asciutta—spaghetti, macaroni, or mostaccioli with Silvia's own tomato sauce—and contorni or side dishes. Gracious touches, such as bright linen napkins and a matching tablecloth that might come with a story from travels to Mexico or India, lovely china, a glass of wine for Paul, and a leisurely demitasse of espresso made me feel Old World civilized in the midst of the rough and tumble of child rearing and starting a career. Yet, I learned that Sunday lunch mirrored ordinary, garden-variety family problems and joys.

At Paul and Silvia's house, our children gravitated to Silvia in the kitchen. All three loved to help her set the lunch table, grate Parmesan cheese, and heap meatballs in a bowl. In their adolescent years, our kids still came along for Sunday lunch to eat the delicious food their grand-mother had prepared but often returned home as soon as they finished, pleading homework. As for John and me, the meaning of Sunday lunches evolved. When we had young children, Sunday lunch was a comfort and support, as Silvia embraced and encouraged not just our children, but also our child rearing. I relaxed because for years, Ellen, Will, and Carol could do no wrong in Paul and Silvia's eyes.

In those early years, John enjoyed sparring with his dad at lunch in friendly political exchanges. Paul commented on Italian affairs, and all of us joined in discussions of state and local happenings. Conversation flew in English for my sake and the children's, although my in-laws preferred Italian in one-on-one conversations with John. I kept my ears open. What I often heard were snippets of tales from life in Italy before Paul and Silvia with John and his sister Luciana as toddlers immigrated to the United States in 1940. Sometimes I pieced together the bits; often the bits shifted or changed over time like the colored shapes in a kaleidoscope.

—w—

That winter day in our home, Paul and Silvia both looked sporty— Paul in a tweed jacket over a navy-blue, V-necked sweater, Silvia in a dark wool skirt with a heavy sweater she had knitted. Anyone looking into our dining room would describe them as a handsome older couple visiting their son and daughter-in-law for an ordinary family gathering. We shared a lunch of lentil soup, hard-crusted bread, and fresh fruit with brownies I'd baked to satisfy Paul's sweet tooth. On that Sunday, no one would have noticed that Silvia, who had learned to drive the same year that John did, drove Paul to our house because Paul had failed a driver's evaluation at Washington University Medical School. The test showed impairment in decision making, traffic awareness, and paying attention. He ran a stop sign. After the test results, Paul handed John his car keys.

The State of Missouri was notified that Paul could no longer drive—effective immediately.

During lunch, John and I chatted with one another, he at one end of our oval table, I at the other. Silvia didn't join the conversation because she could hear neither John nor me in spite of her new hearing aid. Only her tight jaw showed her tension from the previous day. Our old basset hound slept on his quilted bed near Paul, who had greeted him by whispering into his long ears. Paul sat with stooped shoulders, his head over his soup; the hearing aid in his left ear buzzed steadily.

John said to me: "Don't say anything about his hearing aid. It upsets my mom because she blames herself for not being able to take care of him. My dad can't hear the buzz, and he can't fix it anyway."

Head bent to his plate, Paul mumbled something, then laughed to himself. Neither John nor I could divine what he said. Silvia fingered her own hearing aid as if dialing up its volume. She didn't speak to any of us.

We drank espresso, finished the plate of brownies. Our dog barked farewell at the French doors. I missed the Sunday lunches of years past, when we had been guests at Paul and Silvia's. I had felt accepted and loved by John's parents during those brief respites from our child-rearing, career-oriented lives. I couldn't help yearning for those wonderful Sunday meals Silvia prepared when our children were young, when I could relax and let Silvia and Paul take care of all of us.

4

Family Meeting
1996

In the early 1990s, Sharon, a social worker and care manager from a local geriatric consulting firm, gave a talk at my church about recognizing the signs of Alzheimer's disease. I was so impressed with Sharon's knowledge and empathetic handling of this distressing topic that I recounted nearly every detail of her talk to John. I stashed my notes and Sharon's business card in a file. When Paul began to decline markedly in 1993, John hired Sharon to help us sort out how to deal with him. Her firm provided assistance in nursing home placement, medication management, referrals to healthcare agencies, and counseling on a fee-for-service basis. Sharon, a woman in her fifties with clipped blond hair and bright lipstick, served as a social worker for John, his family members, and me as we adapted to our first Alzheimer's patient and as a care manager, guiding us as we learned how to cope with the necessary lifestyle changes associated with the disease.

Though Paul wasn't diagnosed with Alzheimer's disease (to the extent that it can be determined prior to the patient's death) until the winter of 1996, noticeable changes in his behavior and a deterioration of his intellectual capacities pointed toward some form of progressive dementia in 1993, the same year he swam solo in Lake Michigan.

Initially, Sharon spent only a few hours a month with our family. She held one or two monthly counseling sessions with Silvia, sometimes in our living room, so that Paul, who was suspicious of outsiders, would not interrupt or overhear. Thanks to Sharon's advice, John furnished Paul with a Safe Return® bracelet inscribed with his name, an identification number, and the words "memory impaired." Predictably, Paul often refused to wear the bracelet. Sharon also assisted in nursing home choice, consulting with John and me, the initial nursing home selection team.

Sharon's agency charged about $75 per hour in the 1990s. In 2009, care managers like Sharon cost about $100 per hour, billable in increments of 15 minutes. Sharon's help relieved John and me, for we were both still working full time. Sharon's one-on-one counseling sessions with Silvia were covered by Medicare. While Silvia appreciated Sharon's empathetic approach to her caregiving situation, she protested, with her customary independent spirit, that no one could help her. John and I, however, sensed that Silvia felt alone and trapped in a state of constant crisis. As she could do nothing to change Paul's behavior, she thought she was obligated to endure life with her husband no matter how he treated her.

Until Sharon's talk at my church, we had not known that a profession such as hers existed nor how many small, daily alterations of our lives would be required as Paul's condition worsened. John needed, for instance, to redirect his parents' incoming first-class mail to a post office box because Paul seized the mail and lost or hid it. Sharon introduced us to the many Alzheimer's Association services, from family support group meetings to locating dementia nursing units. I availed myself of the Association's free telephone helpline on numerous occasions when an agitated Paul telephoned our house. I often fielded his calls because he knew I prepared my university courses and graded papers at home. Ours was the one telephone number Paul could remember and dial. As I listened to Paul's frequent demands and menaces, knowing that I could call the helpline preserved my equanimity. On the other end of the helpline, a person with a calm voice instructed me in how to respond to my father-in-law with step-by-step suggestions. (See the Resources section at the back of this book for the Alzheimer's Association's toll-free helpline number, as well as its e-mail address, helpful for less urgent concerns and for caregivers who need advice and support.)

John took Silvia to several Alzheimer's Association free support group meetings for caregivers. Even though she was alert to others' tales of Alzheimer's symptoms and progression, Silvia refused to return after attending two or three meetings. She said, "I don't go to sad movies. I don't read sad books. I don't want to go to sad meetings."

Sadness wasn't in the vocabulary of the Silvia I knew. It wasn't that she never felt sad. When she was worried about her son Albert's health, she sat immobile by the swimming pool. She would review, almost obsessively, what she knew of his and his family's life in Washington, D.C. Yet she never called this sadness. Her own emotions were not a topic of discussion; she kept them private and guarded.

But she delighted in her grandchildren with joy lighting her eyes. "Will's going to love this book about Pondus the penguin. Just look at the pictures," she'd said to me. I remember the pages with Pondus in the zoo wearing a red scarf. Or when one grandchild expressed an interest in photography, she rejoiced, "Let me get her a fine camera." Her generosity and insight flowed into action.

Whether she denied the changes in Paul's personality and behavior or was saddened by them, she rarely articulated her feelings to John or to me. I did not ask her or Sharon what the two of them discussed. Nor did John. I recognized a vast generational and cultural divide between us. Silvia would not, as I understood it, reckon head-on with self-analysis or self-pity. Instead, her sadness revealed itself as chair-sitting inertia, an uncharacteristic dullness in her eyes, repeated questions, arthritic pain in her hands, or occasionally even anger. Only by recognizing these signs did I know she was sad.

John collected brochures and fact sheets about the disease, including activities and services provided to families. He and I set about informing ourselves, as if we were once again studying for the legal bar or graduate comprehensive exams. I began to ask several of my friends for advice. Sharon's role was to map the managerial process and cheer us on, even if she could not predict the twists and turns of what can only be called a dread disease.

In December 1996, John came home and said, "Well, it was a parents' day." I knew what that meant and how testy such a day made John and, consequently, me.

"My goddamn father," he began, as he came into the kitchen. "He called me all day long at work. I don't give a flying fuck what he says he needs to do with his stockbroker."

"It must have been bad, John." I empathized because I, too, was receiving calls at my office related to Paul—three in one day when I was grading final exams with a pre-Christmas deadline: the Alumni House inquired about Paul's unpaid bills, a colleague was upset by Paul's late arrival and noisy hearing aid during a lecture, and a friend wondered about Paul's health. Strangers and friends often called me instead of John, I imagined, because of old habits and, though this attitude is changing in the twenty-first century, the belief that caregiving falls within the woman's arena.

Many people apparently thought it was more acceptable to interrupt a woman professor than a male lawyer. Most didn't call Silvia because she had grown defensive and was unable to hear on the phone.

"Bad?" John's voice ricocheted around our kitchen. "You don't get it, how bad it is. I feel like telling him to jam it up his ass!"

"Okay, John, okay."

"Don't okay me. He's not your father."

"I know, I know," I said.

"Next time I'm going to tell him that."

"Just cool it, John. Of course it's tough on you. I get calls about him, too. Okay?"

Neither of us felt at all okay. Since the first of December, our lives, intertwined with Paul's and Silvia's, had been stormy most days.

—⁓—

Sharon warned John, Silvia, Pat, and me that we were moving toward a decision about change, whether it be beefing up help at home or arranging Paul's "placement." Placement meant moving him to a nursing home facility with an Alzheimer's disease unit. One of Paul's doctors noted, "His dementia has progressed to the point that institutional care is appropriate." Paul's aphasia (loss of language) was startling. John knew, however, that his siblings might resist Paul's placement. At Alzheimer's Association briefings for families of the disease's victims, John learned that family members who live out of town often are difficult to convince of the need for action because they cling to views of the victim (usually a parent) from long ago. Out-of-towners, according to the Alzheimer's Association, tend to deny or underestimate the seriousness of the problem. John worked hard to prevent this by keeping Luciana and Albert informed about Paul and Silvia and about Alzheimer's disease. Yet, we had noticed that Paul and Silvia rose to the occasion whenever Luciana or Albert visited, making it harder to persuade them that anything was amiss in their parents' lives. As John broached the topic of placement, he suspected that his sister and brother might be opposed.

We were learning that placement frequently occurs after a "precipitating crisis," which had not happened. Nonetheless, for me, each small crisis felt gigantic, like a "blowout" that set off ripple effects in Paul—physically, emotionally, and psychologically. John and I began to recognize that "plateaus" did follow crises, although plateau is an inaccurate term because it suggests a return to a more reasonable plane. The terms "holding platform" or "pause" are more precise. Alzheimer's disease does not allow a patient to recover or restore rationality. After a crisis, however, the patient may remain on a plateau for days or weeks without a new or convoluted symptom appearing. Inevitably, the patient descends, spiral by spiral, into a Dantean hell.

As family caregivers, we were enmeshed in the daily events on Overhill Drive and blind to how discombobulated our existence was becoming. After each of Paul's blowouts—a frightening wandering episode or a succession of urgent, incoherent phone calls to his broker—Silvia, John, and I experienced our own physical, emotional, and psychological ripple effects. Silvia became more anxious, John grew crankier, and I needed more sleep. All of us were dispirited, desperate for outside intervention. Pat, Silvia and Paul's housekeeper/caregiver, as strong and steady as she was, told me she was exhausted and exasperated with helplessness.

John and I and the entire family were afloat on stormy, uncharted seas with no rudder, no compass. John and I reacted without clearly understanding the extent of Paul's and Silvia's distress. I responded to anguished calls from Silvia about Paul's irrational demands to drive him places, as well as to heartfelt pleas from Pat to do "something," by trying to be a calming influence. Because this was our first go-round with Alzheimer's disease, I trudged through each episode dutifully, without stepping back to get a clearer perspective. I kept up with my academic work and tried to be companionable as I listened to John. He was having a different set of painful experiences with his parents, while handling a full workload and trying to be a supportive husband and son. I was unaware of the deepening strain on the two of us because I coped with each incident reactively, day by day. Gradually, John and I identified ports, like the Alzheimer's Association, for direction and refuge during the storms caused by the early and mid-stages of Paul's disease.

Alzheimer's disease is commonly classified in three stages. John and I realized that we needed to learn the language of the disease, the medical terminology that professionals used when speaking about his father's condition. We needed to understand the vocabulary and the parameters of the disease, even though our experiences with Paul felt much more intense than their dry descriptions. The disease's three primary stages are characterized as (1) mild, when a patient exhibits diminished cognitive and memory functions yet performs acceptably in a familiar routine and environment; (2) moderate, when problems such as wandering and irascibility/anger surface; and (3) severe, when the patient loses most cognitive and memory functions and can no longer perform the activities of daily living (ADLs), such as bathing, toileting, eating, transferring (from bed to chair, for example), dressing, grooming, and hygiene. In the severe third stage of Alzheimer's, a patient usually requires around-the-clock care. (For more details on these stages, consult *The Encyclopedia of Alzheimer's Disease*.)

In the fall and winter of 1996, by the traits we could identify, Paul was beyond the first or mild stage and well into the moderate or mid-stage of the disease. He was on the verge of needing more care than Silvia and Pat could provide. He needed to be placed in a nursing home for Silvia's and our peace of mind. Paul's and Silvia's safety concerned us, too. More serious than the dangers of Paul wandering the neighborhood were those he posed physically toward Silvia. We don't know how often he shoved Silvia, but once he pushed her hard enough that she fell in their tiled bathroom. Paul phoned for help that morning. When I arrived, Paul blocked me from going upstairs to check on Silvia after her "fall."

—∿∿—

That crisis-filled December, our support team included not only Sharon, but also Frances, a family social worker in private practice, whom John and I had consulted off and on over the years. Fifty percent of Fran's hourly fee was covered by my medical insurance through work. Fran had counseled us when our children entered their teens, when they battled over the telephone or use of the car, when they stumbled as they asserted their independence—at times when John and I could not figure out appropriate parental roles. Neither John nor I was used to being introspective or analytical about relationships or emotions. Both of us preferred to act, to live forward. When we realized we were losing our way as parents, Fran had gently prodded us into pausing to look into ourselves. We never dreamed we would call on her to steer us as we attempted to parent our own parents.

A strong woman who loved sports, Fran was fit, alert, and matter-of-fact. I trusted her common-sense approach, her insistence that we hold steady, her careful listening, and her practical wisdom. Her astute questions had lighted our way, causing us to think of more effective ways to cope with our teenagers. And when we consulted her about Paul, her questions helped us clarify the worsening situation.

At one session after John and I had aired our December grievances, Fran stepped in: "John, what will it take for Silvia to let you take over the decision making about your father? Do you and your siblings want to wait for a crisis that your mother can't handle?"

John answered, "Both my siblings think we should wait to move Dad."

Fran came back at him, "Who lives here in St. Louis? What do you think you should do?"

John said, "Maybe I should ask them what they think is best for Mamma?"

"You need to talk to your brother and sister about yourself and the toll that caring for your parents is taking on you." Fran rarely gave such direct advice.

"I need relief, too," I said. I was tense because it was the end of the semester with exams and papers to grade. Dealing with Paul and Silvia exacerbated my usual pre-Christmas anxiety. "I'm rundown. I've nearly had it."

Fran went on, "To live your own lives—that's a reason for placing your father in a nursing home. Your mother's well-being—another reason. You've got to take care of yourselves."

And I whispered, "Amen." But I wasn't sure if I even remembered what taking care of myself meant nor whether I could remember how to go about it. To survive as individuals and to survive as a married couple, we would have to learn to take care of ourselves, to recognize our limits, and to set boundaries. We needed all the help we could find and a bit of protection, too. Fran was an invaluable voice for sanity.

—⁂—

In December 1996, John and I began our weekly Alzheimer-unit search "dates" because Paul had to be moved. After our dates on Saturday afternoons, John and I played tennis—separately—John with a group of men and I with my younger sister, Missy, with whom I relieved my sadness and tension by chatting on our drive to the indoor court and by hitting hard balls. My tall, slim sister, whose legs were even longer than mine, was my favorite tennis rival and listening post. During the previous week, John and I had divvied up a list of homes culled from the yellow pages and friends, nursing homes with names like Bella Villa, Cape Breton Estates, Coach n' Four Place, and Hanley Park. We made calls and set appointments, limiting ourselves to checking out two or three facilities per Saturday. I knew—I guess John did, too—that we'd crumple if we saw more.

We learned the routine. Most Alzheimer's units were locked because patients wander and escape. A receptionist at each nursing home buzzed the unit and pointed the way down a long corridor past pleasant or dozing, often vacuous, patients. Observing us through a peephole, a nurse ushered us in. At each facility, we found ourselves in a scene from a Brueghel painting, full of the moving and the grotesque. Brisk, vigorous walkers attached themselves to our sleeves with pleas to take them home. At one facility, a nurse polished female patients' nails as they sat with blank stares and hands outstretched. A man roamed the halls at another place stark naked. Cries, shouts, and hilarious laughter filled the background as a nurse explained the Alzheimer's "program" and showed us rooms, each one identified by a memory box at the door. A patient's family was asked to fill the box with memorabilia and pictures of the patient in hopes of keeping fresh his or her sense of identity and recognition of self.

We admired gardens with high walls to prevent wandering and a music therapist holding a sing-along of old favorites, such as "You Are My Sunshine." The pacing of walkers and the shouts made discussions feel chaotic, yet almost every staff member at every facility was unflappable in the face of unimaginable doings: a patient constantly banging on a steel fire door, a male patient in a female patient's clothes he had borrowed, and anguished cries of "Take me home." Dante's, Michelangelo's, and Rodin's depictions of hell are no more vivid than these scenes. Inevitably, the head nurse's tranquil voice would rise over this din of vacant, yet vocal humanity: "Be assured that your 'loved one' will be well cared for." Paul, our loved one, we imagined, oh, assured, oh yes, Paul will walk and eat hot pasta and be so carefully attended.

On those Saturdays of searching for a good place for Paul, lunchtime came as a relief. John and I would meet in far-flung malls in west or north St. Louis County, where our choices were fast food or chain restaurants. I was always exhausted by those morning tours, incapable of processing what I'd seen.

"Lordy, lordy, John," I began as I flopped down on a plastic banquette.

"God, Suze. How can we do this to my dad?"

"I need water. Lots of water." My mouth was dry and cracking, as if I'd been on a desert trek.

"All these nursing homes suck." John looked defeated.

"I hate this."

"Me, too. We'd better eat. We'll feel better."

I ate junky foods—fried or greasy or oily. Anything to erase what we'd just seen—a lunch date with pizza on a paper plate with a salad whose dressing I squeezed from an aluminum foil packet or fatty red chili with clumps of an unknown meat. I devoured all sorts of junk food as if I'd run a marathon. It was a horrible yet a precious time for us, as we wondered aloud, even joked about how we ever got to this point in our lives. We had to hold each other up. In that, we could not flinch. Neither of us could fathom this new posture of responsibility for his father and mother. It felt like a nightmare from which we would soon awaken. We tried to convince ourselves to laugh like Figaro (in Pierre Beaumarchais' play, *The Barber of Seville*), who says, "I push myself to laugh from fear of crying."

—⁓—

John's siblings—his younger sister, Luciana, from Massachusetts and his younger brother, Albert, with his wife and two children from near Washington, D.C.—came in 1996 for Christmas at Paul and Silvia's house. Their Christmas visit was annual—the only time every year when John's whole family gathered. Paul and Silvia usually visited Albert and his wife, Lynn, and their children once a year. A gentle man, Albert held a variety of jobs and was involved in childrearing. He had been a volunteer, then a staff member of VISTA (Volunteers in Service to America), he taught little children, and he worked in a college career office. Albert suffered from neurofibromatosis, a serious, often painful condition marked by many neurofibromas, benign tumors that grow in nerve sheaths. Albert and his family were happy to visit with his parents twice a year. Luciana kept in touch with John and shared frequent visits with Paul and Silvia. However, as out-of-towners visiting for annual holiday festivities, Albert and Luciana appeared both to overlook their parents' decline and to rely on John to care for Paul and Silvia.

Following Sharon's advice, we organized a family meeting, including Pat, at our house in front of a crackling fire late one afternoon.

Sharon, as a neutral party and social worker, undertook to run the Christmas meeting in 1996. We had asked our son, Will, to look after Paul while we met.

"So what's going on?" Will asked.

"We've got to decide what to do about your Nonno," John said.

I added, "He can't live at home any more. It's too tough on Nonna."

Will silently watched both of us.

When Will said, "What should I do with Nonno?" he echoed the whole family's dilemma, the uncertainty and the necessary decision.

"He loves to go out. Take him out for hot chocolate," John said.

"This will be the last time, won't it?" Will stated. His hazel eyes, like John's and Silvia's, fixed us both. I read a deep sense of loss behind his quiet composure. Will had always carefully observed others' feelings and interactions. As a child in the first week of elementary school, he sat on the edge of the playground to size up the situation. The friends he chose with careful deliberation remain his friends to this day.

Sharon opened the meeting with a description of Paul's symptoms and the need to move him to a nursing home. Silvia, said Sharon, was unraveling under the pressure of caring for an Alzheimer's patient who was alternately silent, incoherent, wrathful, compliant, dangerous, nasty, sweet, defiant, and loving. In typical Alzheimer's fashion, Paul's internal clock had reset itself so that he often got up and dressed—and for Paul that meant a suit, dress shirt, and a tie—and tried to go out at 3 a.m., then again at 5 a.m. Silvia was frustrated and sleep deprived. Paul was also incontinent and impatient when Silvia and Pat attempted to deal with this condition.

John and I had noticed that Silvia herself was changing, becoming forgetful and cranky. Earlier in the fall, she had exploded, for example, at John and me when John mentioned her hearing loss: "Get out of my house." Silvia had flown at John, her hair and demeanor wild like a witch out of control. John and I had left immediately.

At the family meeting, Sharon laid out the options.

"You can have a team of nurses' aides at your house 24 hours a day every day, or Paul can move to a nursing home."

Silvia spoke first: "When? When can he move?"

"As soon as we can find a male bed," Sharon said. "It may take awhile."

Silvia said, "I can't have people in my house at night."

"Your decision, then?" Sharon asked.

Silvia said, "Paul will have to be moved."

Sharon announced that she and Silvia would visit and choose from three or four homes that John and I had screened on our Saturday dates. The move would occur as soon as a single room became available and the paperwork was completed. Sharon gathered her papers and was gone before we knew it.

After that moment of calm decision, the blood members of the family—John, Luciana, Albert, and Silvia—began to talk and cry and yell all at once. Pat, Lynn, and I watched.

"What will happen to me, to our wonderful house and pool?" asked Silvia.

"Not enough time to consider it," someone shouted.

"It's not fair. . . ."

"What if Sharon isn't really an expert?"

"Who says Papa has Alzheimer's?"

"Why didn't someone tell me this was going on?"

It was the shouts and accusations that I couldn't grasp. I wondered why there were no sobs and moans, memories and sunken shoulders over the plight of this couple—Paul now a wanderer, an aimless wanderer. We should all gnash our teeth and weep for Paul's rapid footsteps, tap-tapping the concrete sidewalks of University City in quest of copies or the mail or a bench where he might alight to dream of his shining Venice. When he spoke of Venice, he called it La Serenissima (the most serene). The sinking city of Venice was sunk deeply in his heart. The city of ancient, cobbled pavements, of piazzas ringing with café voices and the thud of soccer balls, of secret entrances through heavy wooden doors, wrought iron gates, passageways so narrow that they are nearly dark at midday—the city republic known as Venice was the only city Paul's interior compass signaled as home.

I went upstairs to escape. My heart banged in my chest.

Silvia's shrill, angry voice—the agony of quiet, smiling, welcoming Silvia, who never raised her voice when one of my children back-talked or splashed her with a mighty cannonball jump into the pool—rose up our stairs.

My heart pounded. I was miserable. These people in my husband's family were strangers to me in their hot irrationality. I was disgusted by the angry force of John's family that day. Later, as I cleaned up coffee cups, I couldn't stop myself from screaming at anyone who could hear:

"I hate your family, John!"

5

Kaddish in Venice
1997

Early in January, Sharon urged Silvia to implement the family decision about Paul's move. Paul's behavior had worsened. He insisted
on going out late in the evening, and one night he set out in a snowstorm.
Once he woke up and dressed several times during the night, and at 5
a.m. he cooked his own breakfast in preparation for leaving on foot. As
Silvia grew frantic, she could no longer think clearly about a course of
action or about her own self-preservation. One evening John exploded
about Silvia.

"Goddamn it, Suze." I was cooking dinner when John came home
from his office.

"What's going on? Bad day?" It was winter; I was making minestrone
laden with beans and vegetables, my version of Silvia's recipe.

"My mother has got to put her foot down. Refuse to coddle my dad."
John's voice grew louder as his words shot out like a volley of bullets. "He's
a horse's ass, getting up all night long and getting dressed and making

my mom get up. She has to learn to stand up for herself. Not be pushed around."

"Wait, John. She has stood up for herself. Remember about the pistol into the canal?"

When Paul told that story over the years, he showed that he could provoke a challenge and that Silvia with her sharp will could stand up to him.

Paul recounted how he courted Silvia in Venice during the 1930s soon after he had passed the celery-soup test of wills—his versus his future mother-in-law's. Even though he and Silvia became engaged, Paul's visits to the family remained formal by twenty-first century standards.

Before dinner, Paul, still in his officer's uniform, would call at Silvia's family palazzo. Silvia's father remained in his study while her mother installed herself in the high-ceilinged drawing room overlooking the Grand Canal. On John's and my honeymoon to introduce me to his family in Italy, we also visited Silvia's kin. I met Silvia's mother, aged but imposing, on that visit. It was easy to picture her as a grande dame at her needlework as she waited for her children to gather for dinner.

Tall and straight, Paul made an impressive fiancé when he came to call. His military leather shone: his wide belt, his cartridge case, and his pistol holster with its shiny brass snap. When he entered the palace, he handed his hat to Guido and strode across the marble floors as if on parade. He bent gallantly to kiss Silvia's mother's hand and then took up a commanding place in front of the French doors opening onto the balcony above the canal.

One evening Silvia's mother had not yet come down for dinner, but Silvia and her sister, Livia, waited in the drawing room for visitors. When Paul arrived, instead of standing in front of the French doors, he chose a spot between the two girls. With one hand on his hip, he snapped and unsnapped his holster.

That day, without their mother present, the two sisters chatted and whispered together, so the legend goes. Because of the noise of the snap, Livia asked Paul first about the glistening leather of the holster, then about target practice, and at last about the elegant tooling on the pistol handle. Paul brought out his pistol and laid it flat in his palm for her to see. Since the sisters had never seen a gun, they closed in around him to look. The sisters' curiosity about a weapon, forbidden as weapons were in their household, might have seemed almost lascivious. Livia— the brasher, more curious sister—took the gun in her hand. Gingerly at first, she turned it as she traced its silver markings with her fingertip and fondled its oiled butt. In spite of a small measure of curiosity, Silvia averted her eyes and sighed loud in protest, for she was staunch in her antimilitary beliefs.

Just then, Guido ushered in Silvia's mother. Livia quickly returned the pistol to Paul and drew back, leaving Paul bathed in the evening light with his pistol in his outstretched hand. Silvia seized the gun before he could return it to its holster. She pushed aside the gauze curtains at the French doors and threw her suitor's weapon over the balcony into the black water of the Grand Canal.

"Haven't I told you that I hate guns?" Silvia said. I can imagine her pulling up to appear taller than she was, fiery-eyed and absolute in tone.

"I concur," said Silvia's mother. "Much as I am pleased with your calls to my daughters, I am dismayed at your brandishing a pistol in our home."

"But, Mamma," Livia tried to intervene.

"Firearms have no place in our household. Or, for that matter, in civilized society. As you, Paul, and your father are aware, our family has a long tradition of being opposed to the military and to its accoutrements."

Offering Paul his hat, Guido held the door for him as the sisters backed away silently.

The next time Paul came to the palace he wore his uniform and his holster, brightly polished and bearing a new pistol. Silvia's mother was working her needlepoint canvas when he arrived. Her daughters froze in their chairs. Paul stood silhouetted before the doors; he snapped and unsnapped the gun's holster. Silvia smiled brightly at her handsome husband-to-be. Her mother lifted her head, her eyes piercing and her needle menacing.

With unusual irony, Paul always remarked that he never again took out his pistol in Silvia's family salon. Silvia cited this tale as her first and most spectacular anti-war action—a precursor of her lifelong, unwavering stance.

—⁓—

"Wait a moment," I said. "I thought you'd decided to move your dad? What's the deal this time?"

"We can't move him yet because no male room is available. Last night the whole night he was up. Then my mom calls me at work. She has to learn to control my dad, get a grip. Tell him to shape up. I don't give a fuck what my dad tells my mom to do. And I yelled at her to take matters into her own hands." He yelled at me, at the stove, at the simmering soup, at the four walls of our kitchen.

"John, she's an 84-year-old woman who's not getting enough sleep and who has her own ways of dealing with your dad. True, she rarely stands up to your dad these days." Taming Paul with Alzheimer's was not as simple as throwing his gun into the Grand Canal.

"Don't give me that bullshit. She's got to take charge. Stop my dad." And on and on—until John spent his anger and frustration at his own inability to resolve this untenable situation. This was a John I barely recognized.

I let the fragrance of our soup lift me away—its carrots, onions, thyme, and bay leaf—away from John's voice bouncing against our kitchen cabinets. We'd sat on a terrace in Burgundy drinking a sweet red Kir with the same smells of a long-simmering stew behind us. It was in the 1970s; John and I were following a medieval pilgrimage route of Romanesque churches—squat in their stone sturdiness, intriguing with carved column capitals. Alone together on our first European trip since our children's births, we savored slow, spill-free meals. I could still taste a chicken and cream dish; I felt the uneven paving stones in cool churches under my feet; I thought of those companionable hours we'd saved for in our intense child-rearing years. The angry swearing of this person named John reverberated in our kitchen. How, when would this end? When could we sit next to each other in a town square, reveling over the daily life of a French town unfolding before us? When would John's cursing at last give way to "Can you believe the light, Suze, the way it falls on that tile roof across the way?"

Our soup was ready. We ate it and drank wine together. I hoped the phone wouldn't ring that evening, just that one evening, because I felt depleted. John's outbursts—understandable as they were—left me worn and limp. My heart went out to him in this Alzheimer's trap where he was caught. Out to us. Out to myself as I wondered when this terrible time would be over.

—⁂—

By the middle of January, it felt as if we were on borrowed time with Paul and Silvia. Pat maintained the shell of an orderly daytime routine at their house. Paul frequently got up and wandered through the house at night. He could easily start venturing outside and into the streets. We feared he might hurt Silvia if she tried to stop him. We had narrowed our nursing home search to several with dedicated Alzheimer's units—locked secure facilities with specially trained staff. The problem was availability of a single room for a male. For several days in my office at lunchtime, I called each nursing home, inquiring about the availability of a bed for Paul.

The toll on John was evident. Even after a pleasant Sunday lunch with Paul and Silvia, a bedraggled John slept for two hours in the afternoon.

On Silvia's 85th birthday in January, we were ebullient because, according to Silvia, Paul had gone out to buy her flowers. The next day, Pat recounted that the flowers created a firestorm. In fact, Paul had left the house alone without saying where he was going. Pat followed Paul in her car as he walked in a snowy street to Clayton, a nearby business district. He refused to get into her car. A policeman helped, coaxed Paul into Pat's car, and followed them home. Pat and Paul purchased the flowers later.

As potentially dangerous situations came closer and closer together, Sharon repeated that it was time "to intervene." She again called a meeting with Silvia, John, and me at our house while Paul stayed at home with Pat.

I had heard the family legend of an intergenerational meeting at Silvia's parents' summer house in Cortina in 1938. That summer of 1938, Paul and Silvia, with their babies, John and Luciana; Silvia's older sister, Livia, and her husband; and Silvia's mother vacationed at the family villa in Cortina, north of Venice in the Italian Dolomite Mountains. Guido, the butler who had stoically served Paul "celeries" in his soup, became the chauffeur, driving some family members, including the family cook, from Venice.

The cook, a stolid, silent woman with steel-gray hair bound like wires into a bun, ruled the Cortina kitchen, as she did the one in Venice. No one else in the family participated in kitchen activities. In my imagination I picture a cook who produced her own pastas, using strong shoulders to roll lengths of lasagna noodles. She pounded pinkish-white veal into thin leaves for scallopini and dusted wild mountain raspberries with powdered sugar for dessert. While she surveyed the family, dining under the mountain pines in the garden, she stood in the kitchen doorway with her feet apart, her arms akimbo, heavy with pride in her culinary creations. This strong woman was quick, lightning quick, with her bare right hand. John told me she could snatch a fly from the air, any fly that dared to venture past her into the kitchen. John and his cousins, who spent several post-war summers at the villa, marvel to this day at the cook's fly-catching prowess. Nary a blink, a shoulder twitch, just an arm shooting forth, her fingers plucking the victim from the summer air. So tight was her squeeze that the fly dropped dead as the cook opened her palm for it to fall at her feet.

One summer day in 1938, Silvia walked into the cook's kitchen with pen and notebook in hand. The cook, so the family tale went, was preparing risotto, the slow-cooking rice that needs constant stirring as it absorbs cups of chicken broth.

"Here I am," Silvia announced, "to learn how to cook." In her mid-twenties, Silvia had shiny black hair in flat waves and flashing hazel eyes that gave her a spirited look. Her animated eyes often spoke her emotions more than words; she was considered the shy one in her family.

"Why in the world?" said the cook without looking up from stirring the broth.

"Because I want to learn what goes into risotto, step by step. I ought to be able to cook it myself."

"I don't know until I begin to prepare it."

"Stop and think what you use. Please." Silvia's voice was pleading.

"Just this time so that I can write it down."

"Follow me as I gather up what I need," the cook grumbled.

Silvia followed the cook from one cabinet to another. Leaning with her over a bin of rice, Silvia counted the handfuls the cook threw into a deep skillet with hot olive oil. Next she shook the rice, then began to stir in a cup of boiling chicken stock. Silvia gauged how much salt the cook measured in the well of her palm and watched her sprinkle threads of saffron into the bubbling rice. Silvia wrote an approximation of quantities in her notebook.

Over the weeks that August, while she collected recipes for everyday dishes, she asked for cooking terms. As I envision the drama building, Silvia grew more persistent.

"Would you say that the fruit is marinating or macerating in the wine?"

"Why, why, why does it matter?" The cook grew impatient. "Silvia, you're asking too many questions." In the kitchen, the cook took on imperious airs: "Simply leave the fruit in the wine for a few hours."

"Frying or sautéing—which are you doing to that eggplant?"

"Words, Silvia, words." The cook shook the skillet. The purple-skinned vegetable sent pops of oil into the air. "Watch if you must, but stand back. You're never going to have to cook."

"I want to know how. More than that: I want some recipes written down."

The cook muttered, "Why do you need so many details?"

"Because I need details and numbers in the recipes, for keeping in touch when we leave."

"When who leaves?" The cook stopped chopping zucchini. "To go where?"

"Most of us. Before long. Guido will explain. It's because of Mussolini and Hitler. The racial laws and the way they're treating Jews."

The cook dropped her knife on the counter, picked it up and wiped the blade on her apron. Staring hard at Silvia, she said in clipped phrases, "Watch the pasta. Don't let it boil. Turn the heat down, Silvia. Grate the cheese."

"Where's the grater? How much do I need?"

"Haven't you been watching?"

"I'm going to use recipes when we write to each other," Silvia said as she scraped a block of hard Parmigiano-Reggiano cheese against the grater. "I'll show you the system I have in mind."

With a long wooden fork, the cook poked the pasta. Beads of sweat burst out on her forehead. "Your family has never bothered anyone."

"Paul's job at the university isn't safe. It's all just beginning. Is this enough cheese?" Silvia asked.

"Put the cheese in the pasta. Add some oil. Then stir it to see. Who is leaving?"

"It looks perfect now, doesn't it?" Silvia stirred with the wooden fork. "Paul and I and the children. My brothers—Mario to Argentina and Bruno to France, then on to the United States. My mother and father should leave, although they don't believe there's anything to worry about. Can't you guess at how much oil and cheese I've added?"

"Judge for yourself. Next week, we'll try something more difficult. I'll go slowly so that you can write it down." The cook shuffled away, "Get on out of the kitchen. The others will be home from hiking. I have to finish up."

The next evening after Guido lit the hurricane lamps in the garden and Silvia's mother wrapped herself in a black-fringed shawl against the cool mountain air, Silvia convened her family. "Hush everyone. We need to have a plan to keep in touch somehow if we're separated. That's why I have been learning to cook."

Her mother cleared her throat and said, "There won't be any problems."

Silvia looked boldly at her mother, "We need a system that we agree
on now. We're going to use recipes. Ordinary ones. Just women doing
their usual cooking exchanges."

Silvia's sister, Livia, drummed her fingers on the table, "I don't know
any recipes. Besides, I'm not leaving Italy."

"Look them up in a book. Get the cook to give you some. It doesn't
matter whether the recipe works. No one will censor recipes mailed
between women."

Silvia's mother cleared her throat again. Her hands came out from
under her shawl and rested on the edge of the table. The fringe of the
shawl spread out toward her daughters like fingers grasping. She said,
"Nobody will bother us. For more than four hundred years, no one has
bothered us. You, Silvia and Paul, are overreacting. And you, too, Livia,
what with your taking your family out to the farm to stay."

"Don't start that now, Mother," Livia said.

"It's different this time," said Paul. "It is very dangerous."

I had gleaned the details of this family meeting, of this homespun
mode of communication and of family self-preservation in this perilous
moment. Some details came from Silvia, some from Luciana, and, of
course, some from my imagination fired by John's and my visit to the
villa in Cortina—now an inn. I had tried to summon up how a code
with recipes might work. No one in the family knew. Silvia's first recipe
from the cook—the one for risotto—would have been the opening tool
for communication. We all agreed that a recipe for pasta frolla, the family's favorite butter cookie with jam in the center, would have traveled
across the seas. Family members succeeded in keeping in touch. Some-

how, Silvia received assurance that her parents were safe in Switzerland after hiking over the Alps. Once the war was over, Silvia's parents moved back to Italy and settled in Rome, while maintaining the villa in Cortina where John, his family, aunts, uncles, and cousins gathered several times in the 1950s.

No one in the family remembered to ask Silvia or her sister or mother how the recipe code worked, nor has any one of the younger generation been able to reconstruct how it carried news.

—m—

Practiced and calm, Sharon repeated the issues demanding intervention at our January meeting, which would again fracture John's family: 1) Paul's unreasonable demands. Silvia could not meet them. Nothing would satisfy Paul. 2) Paul's bad temper. Silvia was always anxious and tired. 3) Paul's wandering. He had neither impulse control nor judgment. He could no longer think through the consequences of his actions or words. 4) Paul's getting up at night. Now he slept during the day. 5) Paul's bladder incontinence.

These problems, said Sharon—personality changes, irritability, wandering, reversed biological clock, incontinence—were typical of middle stage Alzheimer's disease. And these symptoms were more than Silvia, at 85, could be expected to deal with. Although John's siblings had agreed to placement for Paul at our December meeting, after they returned home, they contended that John and I had exaggerated. Indeed, Paul and Silvia had pulled themselves together and acted rather normal during their Christmas visit. I had learned that this ability to rise to an occasion and mask symptoms is typical of Alzheimer's patients, as is family members' denial of the disease. As the book, *Mayo Clinic on Alzheimer's Disease*, points out, "Denial is a natural reaction to painful news and can be a form of protection in difficult situations. . . . Family members in denial may question your judgment and discourage you from using essential resources" (164).

With her outsider's credibility, Sharon pushed forward: "The situation is at an intolerable level." She reiterated, as in December: "You are at the point of either needing around-the-clock help or placement."

Silvia said she could not tolerate around-the-clock caregivers in her home. We needed to find a nursing home for Paul immediately. We worried about Silvia alone in her big house with Paul at night. Silvia asked Pat to increase her hours until Paul's placement, as Pat was a stabilizing presence especially at the end of the day, when Paul would "sun-down." The term "sun-downing" describes disruptive evening behavior, including increased confusion and demands for constant attention, typical of those with Alzheimer's.

In late February, I went to Stanford University in California on academic business. I participated in a brainstorming session about preparing Ph.D. candidates to teach in higher education, an arena in which I had done research and created programs with my graduate students at Washington University. I was interested in this exchange with colleagues from around the country who were doing similar work, and I needed a respite from parent troubles. When I came home, we celebrated John's 60th birthday with his parents, who came to our house for dessert. Silvia reported a visit with Pat to the orthopedic doctor because of some pain in her hip. The doctor found her fine except for a tad of arthritis in that hip.

—⁘—

The arthritis was a reminder of the broken hip Silvia suffered in Rome when she was in her mid-seventies, ten years ago. Silvia's practical bent manifested itself in large, squashy nylon handbags that she favored for trips to Italy. When she found the perfect model, Silvia bought several identical ones. The model came in tan, sturdy nylon with canvas webbing shoulder straps and multiple zippered pockets, including a hidden inside pouch. Silvia packed the handbag with a flashlight; a glasses repair kit; sun and reading glasses; bottled water; an address book; toiletries; separate leather cases for passports, credit cards, travelers checks, and Italian currency; and stationery items for postcards the Italian family signed around the lunch table and sent home to us in the States. She also needed to carry a lightweight shawl and a small pair of binoculars. She probably packed a roll of duct tape, too. So spacious was the bag that Paul importuned Silvia to tote his guidebooks, extra glasses, and keys. Silvia would shift this cumbersome load first to one shoulder, then to the other during a day of sightseeing.

On a summer day in Rome, Silvia, Paul, and another couple climbed down from a tour bus. Silvia must have been the last in line to descend behind the other three. A Vespa roared close to the group. Its driver stretched out an arm and grabbed Silvia's tan nylon bag and tried to speed away. But Silvia did not let go of it. She held on while the robber gunned the Vespa's motor to escape. To wrench the handbag from her strong hands, the thug knocked Silvia down to the pavement and rode off with it before the others realized what was happening. She was rushed to a nearby hospital, where a surgeon placed pins in her broken hip. Purchases on Silvia's credit cards showed up through the length of Italy for luxury goods, such as women's shoes and leather purses.

In St. Louis, Silvia's doctor counseled her to take care of her bones, noting some osteoporosis. She began taking a calcium supplement and eating more dairy foods. John's sister, Luciana, sent a yogurt maker and the culture needed for the first batch. Tidy and straightforward, the machine sat on a kitchen windowsill, where Silvia plied it with the ingredients to make a thick yogurt she flavored with the summer fruit she loved. But gadgets—and there were many over the years—came in and often went out of favor with Silvia. Some she clung to forever, such as the padded garden kneeler with handles to help her stand up after weeding and the gripper to facilitate opening jars. But the yogurt maker waned as Silvia's hip healed. And her bones—alas—took a back seat to photography and the basement darkroom she built for herself.

Soon after her hip healed, Silvia took up photography seriously. First, she enrolled in a course at a local college where the professor—an Italian by birth—encouraged and stimulated her creativity. Then, with a few others who had taken the course, she formed a photography group that met regularly to critique one another's work.

Silvia basked in her newfound passion. She was transformed by having an expertise all her own, one where her eye for architectural detail revealed itself. I had always known Silvia could design things. She had drawn the plans that tucked a swimming pool into an improbable wedge of property beside their house. With its teardrop shape, the pool defied architects and designers who had insisted that there was not enough space. Yet, she made it fit. With duct tape and lots of ingenuity, Silvia fabricated sturdy repairs as well as jerry-built contraptions in her garden. She combined these talents and remodeled a basement room into a darkroom, mastered the chemistry of developing and printing, and produced black-and-white photos of buildings and people in faraway places like Uzbekistan, where she and Paul had traveled.

Silvia proudly spread prints on the dining room table for us to study after a Sunday lunch.

"I think the background could be lighter. The contrasts aren't right. What do you think?" Silvia asked.

"Can you see that tile work up there on the dome? It's fantastic, isn't it?"

We compared her prints, offered commentary, asked for architectural information, and admired the decorative features she singled out in her work. Silvia, at 76, invented an artistic kingdom in a cool, dark basement room that smelled of chemicals—pure magic!

And magic enough that she and several others held a group exhibition under the tutelage of their photography teacher. Silvia chose photos mostly of architectural details, such as roof trim or light falling at an unexpected angle on the face of a building. A few included people in markets or crouched by a doorway in an exotic place she and Paul had visited. She gave each photo a matter-of-fact title, like "Kremlin, Moscow," which scarcely did justice to the glittering domes with intricate crosses captured high against a cloudless sky. Her signature, Silvia Rava, was barely visible in the corner.

I had never seen Silvia put herself forward this way. At the opening of the exhibition, she wore a purple wool suit, her white hair brilliant in contrast. For once, she—not Paul—greeted people and received compliments. With pleased modesty, she inclined her head to smile as praise came her way.

During the years when photography filled Silvia's time, she abandoned the calcium supplements and ate a hunk of cheese or supermarket yogurt for lunch. Formal therapy or exercise that might have held her osteoporosis at bay went by the boards. Later, the osteoporosis caused her to limp and curved her spine into a dowager's hump, which thrust her head forward like a bird seeking food.

—⁂—

At 7:15 a.m. on the first day of my Washington University spring break in 1997, Paul telephoned. He needed us right away, something about Silvia, who had fallen in the night and couldn't walk or move because of insufferable pain in her arthritic hip. I rode with her in an ambulance

to Jewish Hospital, where X-rays were taken. It took John, Pat, and me
to oversee Paul and Silvia at the hospital. Paul wandered away; I was in
charge of him. John talked to doctors while Pat held Silvia's hand. Silvia
was admitted, then released the next day. The diagnosis was an arthritis
attack in her once-broken hip.

Paul's and Silvia's difficulties escalated. I asked friends with Alzheimer's-afflicted parents—one with a mother who hammered down a door,
another whose mother climbed over the high wall of a nursing home
garden—what lay ahead. I asked how they coped because I believed if
I knew, I could prepare. Maybe I would begin to do scientific research,
just as I was trained in literary scholarship. I could read, make notes,
and hypothesize, based on my findings and my observations about what
would come. A reliable scientific narrator might reveal what lay ahead.
It didn't take much inquiry for me to grasp that Alzheimer's disease is
unreliable and untidy and that the greatest stress and damage would be
to Silvia as Paul's caregiver. Paul would continue on. I was resigned to
more crises, numb.

To ease my numbness, I went to church regularly. During silent
prayers, I implored God to help me. Yet, I didn't know what the nature of
help would be. I knew the joys and sustenance of girlfriends: I walked on
Thursdays with my dear friend from the days we rode the bus to school
together in seventh grade. In retrospect, I apologize to her for the monologues of frustration I delivered as we covered city block after block with
our dogs. They were monologues about late-night phone calls from John's
parents, about Paul's incessant demands on John. Several women and I
went out for dinner every other month; we made a rule of no more than
ten minutes of whining about family—children, parents, grandchildren,
partners, or spouses. Wine and tapenade quickly lightened our spirits
and changed our focus. John and I stuck together tightly, fully aware that

we needed to make time for dates; to continue planning, training for and taking hiking trips to different places every year—the French Alps in 1996, the Tetons, and the Canadian Rockies; to be tender and ever-forgiving with each other's ill temper or numbness.

—⁓—

My mom's 85th birthday fell on the day Silvia was released from the hospital, adding a good moment to the bad moments with John's parents. Missy and I gave Mom a birthday lunch at Missy's house. Mom chose eight friends who were her contemporaries as guests. It took heroics for these women to get out, even using canes. They walked tentatively up Missy's driveway and along the uneven path into her sunny house. Mom's lifelong friend, Madeline, had skin as thin as waxed paper, stretched over delicate facial bones. When she spoke in her soft voice about the Japanese drawings she had collected and studied over a lifetime, her face looked as if it were lit from within. Patricia, a single woman who held an important job at a nonprofit agency, wore short white gloves and gave Mom mono-grammed linen handkerchiefs. Stella, a retired art museum educator with a gravelly voice, wore a bright yellow jacket over a black and white polka dot outfit. Around the lunch table, we discussed everything—theater in St. Louis, museums, politics, and Katharine Graham's autobiography. That Saturday at lunch, I welcomed this affirmation of life for 80-year-olds as a counterbalance to the tension of Paul and Silvia's existence.

—⁓—

When a male bed became available at one of our nursing home choices in late March 1997, we scheduled Paul's move for early April. Luciana agreed to come to St. Louis. Albert telephoned to plead with us to postpone the move, to reflect further. John and Luciana went forward. Two days prior to the move, Silvia fell and broke her pelvis while shopping for underwear for Paul: a scene like getting a kid ready for camp.

Before she reported her fall to the doctor, she insisted on packing Paul's bags with his newly purchased and labeled underwear. Silvia's doctor hospitalized her, then scheduled a stay in a rehabilitation center. Because Silvia had repeatedly articulated her desire not to live in her house alone, she would move into an "independent" apartment in a retirement center in St. Louis. John and Silvia had long ago agreed on this plan and had reserved a unit with a deposit.

On April 4, Luciana flew from Boston to help us move Paul to the nursing home. John orchestrated the move. Paul knew nothing. While Silvia was in the hospital, Pat moved Paul's clothing and some books and photos to the nursing home, where she arranged his simple single room. The Alzheimer's unit Paul went to discouraged families from bringing many personal furnishings because Alzheimer's patients lose their sense of boundaries and possessions, using one another's clothes, toiletries, and glasses.

On moving day, John and I joined Luciana at breakfast time at Paul and Silvia's house. Pat had arrived early, helped Paul with breakfast, and given him a dose of a calming medication prescribed by the nursing home. The four of us—Luciana, John, Pat, and I—were ready to insist on the move if Paul should resist. John and Luciana had planned a script to inform him. John would announce matter-of-factly that he was going to take Paul on an outing. Then he and Luciana would set out with Paul. Pat and I would clean the breakfast dishes and straighten the house. When we made these plans, Pat had asked for a week off to recover. Luciana would return to Boston. And I would leave to teach my classes at the university.

"Papa," John began, sitting at the kitchen table as Paul drank his coffee, "I came over this morning to take you on an outing."

It sounded flatly routine: father and son mapping the day ahead, coffee brewing, dishes clinking in the sink, April birds singing in Silvia's pink dogwood tree next to the pool. A grand day for an excursion.

"Oh," Paul said. "I'd better get my coat."

"You can finish your coffee before we leave." John was caught off guard by his father's readiness to go out.

"And I will need my wallet."

"It's here, Papa," said John. Forewarned of the need to maintain the identity conferred by a wallet, John had filled an old one of Paul's with an expired AAA membership card, a car wash coupon, and five $1 bills.

Luciana said brightly, "We're all ready then."

"You're off," Pat added.

Paul put the wallet in his trouser pocket, slipped on his coat, and tucked the morning paper under his arm—everyday gestures, voices even, car humming, off they went, away from everything Paul and Silvia had constructed in their new country, off to the never-never land of people whose brains had grown so tangled and scrambled and muddled that the simple gesture of donning a coat and picking up a newspaper came to seem privileged and perfect, for those ordinary gestures soon evolved into the odd, the jerky, the random, the violent, and the repetitive pinches, parries, bites, and scratches of a very sick Alzheimer's patient.

John and Luciana broke down in tears when the heavy doors of the Alzheimer's unit locked behind their father. Their parents were now being cared for by others. Paul and Silvia's house was full of things but not people. Over the next few months, Luciana and Albert came to St. Louis to help us empty the house of its contents. Eventually the house was sold.

The Alzheimer's unit staff recommended that Paul's family not visit for at least two weeks after placement. This allowed Paul, they alleged, to make the separation and to adapt to his new surroundings. Thus, when the family did visit, the theory was that the patient would no longer be tempted to leave. All this would happen in only two weeks after a lifetime in the world. I was silently incredulous. They told us that during this time, family members would have adjusted, rested, and perhaps restored themselves to be ready for the "placement" phase of an Alzheimer's patient's deterioration. After they began to visit their loved one, families were advised not to take the patient away from the facility, at least patients like Paul, who was physically strong, willful, and capable of "escaping."

After John's first visit to his father in the nursing home, he declared, "My dad is fitting in with life among the lesser animals."

At the beginning of his placement, Paul relished a bath in a large machine in a communal bathing room. Shaped like a diving bell, the tub and its seat tipped as it filled with warm water. In this bathosphere, Paul must have felt for a second as if he were swimming again in his teardrop-shaped pool designed by Silvia or floating in the limpid Adriatic at the Lido, where he spent many an August. But in one of the curious twists of Alzheimer's disease, he lost his taste for the tub, lost his desire for any sort of bathing. No coax, bribe, or demand seemed to work until a nurse appealed to John to intervene. How would that go? Father and son stripped naked, lathering up in the shower together? Instead, somehow John cajoled Paul into getting undressed. John rolled up his sleeves, took off his shoes, leaned into the shower, and turned on the water. He invited his father in as he shook the drops of water from his forearms. John felt as if he were an intrepid adventurer as he undertook this caregiver role. Innocent, neither he nor I ever imagined that Alzheimer's disease and caring for an Alzheimer's patient meant abandoning all expectations and conventions about parent-child relations. I wondered if John had ever seen his father fully naked.

On a balmy June day, John reported that while he and Paul sat in the walled garden at the nursing home, his father looked at him and said, "After everything that I've done, I'm reduced to this?" Sporadic lucidity—therein lay the dismal irony of this scourge of a disease.

Late in June 1997, John and I took a holiday to Seattle to see our younger daughter, Carol, and her fiancé, Noel. Between two weekends of visiting them, our plan was to hike in the rainforest, along the coastal tidewaters, and in the mountains on the Olympic Peninsula.

At the end of our first day in Seattle, we returned to our bed and breakfast inn after touring the historic underground city to find multiple pink slips—phone messages with the URGENT box checked on each one. Paul had been removed from his nursing home because he had punched a visitor and shoved an aide. Because of his strength and unpredictability, he was considered a danger to others. So he was moved to the geriatric psychiatric section of a major hospital in St. Louis. Silvia was unable to cope with any medical decision making about Paul. The doctors would attempt to find appropriate medications to stabilize Paul's behavior—an effort that turned out to take about one month of hospitalization.

In order to confer with doctors after their early morning rounds and because of the two-hour time difference between the Pacific Northwest and St. Louis, John began each Olympic Peninsula vacation day making calls at 6:30 a.m. I would roll over in bed and watch him pace outdoors with a cordless phone in one hand, the other hand gesticulating emphatically as he consulted with medical staff. Framed by towering Norfolk pines and Douglas firs, John looked very small.

—⁂—

In early October, John was so preoccupied with each of his parents that he talked nonstop about them. John and I became Silvia's whipping posts, as she lashed out because she'd been moved from her beloved house with its swimming pool and garden, even though the move was a choice she had knowingly made years before. Doctor's orders that she no longer drive magnified her loss of independence and her anger with us as "enforcers." Her loss of Paul to a nursing home left her alone without her lifelong partner. Even though Paul had been terribly difficult to live with for the past few years, Silvia missed his physical presence. We both understood not to take Silvia's frequent outbursts personally.

Never self-pitying, John was worn out and drained. He poured out his anguish about the minutiae of the daily grind of parent care, wrapping all his emotions in anger. Listening to John at the end of each day, I, too, was drained. I was faltering. I wanted to shake my fist at the God to whom I politely prayed on Sunday mornings.

A pamphlet we received from the Alzheimer's Association announced courses for caregivers on "how to cope." It recommended authors Mace and Rabins' "bible" for Alzheimer's families, called *The 36-Hour Day*, which we borrowed immediately from the Alzheimer's Association library.

After Paul's medications controlled his violent striking out, he moved to an Alzheimer's unit in a university-affiliated nursing home some distance from Silvia's apartment. As the days grew shorter that fall and the weather colder, Pat drove Silvia to visit Paul less often. At the nursing home, everyone seemed cooperative: the nursing staff asked for a scrapbook of everyday activities with the Italian words that Paul was used to. Paul agreed to take his many medications as long as a nurse embedded them in ice cream. All day each day he paced the halls and greeted people with as much grace and charm as he had exuded most of his life. He lost his glasses, his hearing aids, his false teeth, and many of his clothes, not because he had set them aside for a swim in Lake Michigan. Instead, sartorial precision no longer mattered. We once found him wearing women's pajamas, mismatched socks, and a bathrobe in broad daylight, and one night wearing dress shoes while lying in bed under the covers. Yet, with true bonhomie, he introduced John to anyone around as "mio figlio, my son."

Paul had always been an accomplished greeter. At his fiftieth wedding anniversary party, he had inclined his head and kissed a guest's hand. He offered in his enchanting Italian accent, "You look lovely tonight," as his lips brushed the back of the woman's hand. Clearly, this woman, like many others, believed him. Numerous women in the past had fallen for Paul's charming wiles.

While he didn't learn men's shoulder-slap greetings, Paul worked hard on idiomatic English. Sports terms, especially from baseball, were a must in the male-dominated litigation world where he practiced law. Yet it was difficult for an urbane Venetian who claimed to know how to row a gondola to assimilate the parlance of locker rooms or baseball broadcasts. When John was young, Paul enlisted a colleague to take John to the Cardinals' home baseball games so his son could learn about the sport and its lingo. Those outings as well as evenings listening to Harry Caray on a small radio turned John into a Cardinals fan. To this day, John remembers myriad baseball statistics and counts his collection of 1940s baseball cards as treasure. "For one of my grandsons," he says, if I ask about the future of the cards.

For Paul, while the language of baseball remained elusive, his attempts to try expressions in conversations with me made the two of us laugh in our shared flair for language games. One Sunday at lunch, he described an encounter with a woman at a cocktail party: "She was very charming. I struck right out with her."

I raised my eyebrows: "Oh, I'm so sorry. How did that happen?" I thought I'd string Paul along.

Paul wrinkled his high forehead. "Am I confused, Susan? Why are you sorry? Maybe it's . . . I'm confused."

"Was it a good or bad encounter?" I asked mock seriously.

"Do I mean to say I struck up something with her?"

We played with that over our pasta—strike out, now what exactly does that mean? And with a woman? Strike up—is that from baseball or a marching band? Then how do you strike up a conversation? Strike back is fight talk. What about a lucky strike? Or getting to first base or stealing second or rounding third? And what to do if the judge asks about your batting average or the three-strikes-and-you're-out rule?

"Susan," Paul asked me one day when Alzheimer's already had a grip on him, "What is the difference between a university president and a university chancellor? Which one would be the head at a university like Padua?"

Had Paul at last reached his own late 1930s story in the autobiographical opus? He had appeared to be stuck in the late 1920s and early 1930s. Would he put down on paper the story of how his sister-in-law—a savvy and glamorous Austrian Jew who'd seen what Hitler had done to Jews in her country—had warned him about the Nazis? The family was gathered in the Dolomites at their villa. At one meal, the sister-in-law announced, "We're going to have to leave our home." Soon after, Silvia called her family meeting to present the recipe code. Later that very autumn, the fascists posted their sign on the university door at Padua.

"I talked to an important person that day in 1938 to be sure I understood the sign. Was it the chancellor or the president, Susan?"

I wanted with all my heart to help Paul recapture those memories, those stories that would explain how he'd arrived in this dining room in our city with his family when I was just a child. I promised to check on the Italian university hierarchy with a colleague at my university. But when I came back to Paul with an answer, the question had evaporated. Paul's focus had floated off and would be that way until the end.

My last "conversation" with Paul took place with the two of us sitting at a table in his spare, single room at his second nursing home about one month before he died.

To provide some bit of stimulation, some tidbit from his past, I took Paul several picture books of Venice—the handsome, glossy ones that feature photos of St. Mark's Square full of pigeons or flooded in late autumn or shrouded with fog that mutes the porticoes and makes the Campanile di San Marco vanish. The books always show gondolas, the Bridge of Sighs, the Rialto Bridge, and a secret piazza with small boys in shorts kicking around a soccer ball. So familiar were these sights that Paul would feel soothed and reconnected to his native land—that was what I imagined. They might even unlock some language with meaning, I thought, in that era before I'd lived through multiple Alzheimer's cases.

With the book flat on the table, he and I turned pages as I narrated from picture titles and memory. Dressed this time in a white shirt with tie and suit trousers, Paul sat on the edge of his chair, attentive like a school child. To what? My voice? My body or John's? Warm family surrounding him? The pictures, a voice within himself, or nothing? Maybe at this almost silent, yet still mobile, stage of Alzheimer's, Paul's mind merely was an engine pushing him to pace the hallways of the nursing home, to swallow the strawberry ice cream laced with his medications. Walking, swallowing, greeting others—Paul was a shell of the man who had had the insight and courage to remove his family from Italy, where they had long been established as an upper-middle-class family of Jewish merchants integrated into Venetian society.

I paused at a picture of St. Mark's Square—black and white, only a few people about; the shadows thrown by street lamps at the edge of the cobblestones suggested twilight.

"Splendid, isn't it?" I mused idly.

"I have to hurry now," Paul answered. I can't remember whether he spoke in Italian or English, although he spoke primarily Italian by this time. I would have answered him in my own pidgin Italian.

"Ah," I said, not knowing whether to turn the pages or wait for Paul's answer. He jumped in.

"They're waiting for me, the soldiers. I need to save it. Venice."

"You and the soldiers?"

"I have to move on. It's important. With the soldiers. And saving it." Paul's voice was agitated. The right knee that he bounced as if it were inhabited by an independent genie began to bounce. John and Luciana both bounced with the same nervous tic, like a genetic hangover from an unconquerable anxiety that demanded mindless motion for comfort.

I wasn't sure what the photo awakened nor where it might take us, this Venetian gentleman, whose mind had abandoned him and set him adrift in a fragmented landscape with words popping out like gremlins from behind trees, and me. It was a forest, I imagined, where he wandered as snatches of the Italy of his past and the names for his life's happenings hung randomly like the last leaves in November's woods. Out of reach.

"May I turn the page, Paul?"

"Please hurry."

Why should Paul hurry? There is a line in *Alice in Wonderland* when the White Rabbit mutters to himself about hurrying. The Paul I had known had hurried enough now. This Paul, as I perceived him, had been on a long chase to save, not Venice, but himself. Luciana saw Paul as chasing after a dream we called America—freedom, equality—in his valiant and seminal work on the St. Louis school desegregation case. But his chase, to me as a daughter-in-law, looked more convoluted, more deeply personal than such ideals. The profound, unspoken sorrow over his mother's death in his early years demanded all his power to chase away, a lifelong sadness he had masked with cheer and cleverness. He had mustered all his considerable wits to chase that pain.

Nor could Paul hurry past the memory of his own misunderstanding of the fascist threat in Italy. This old man, dignified enough to present his son to the nursing staff on each visit, this old man, once a dashing chap of prowess and promise, had joined the Italian fascist movement, as had his father. When the movement turned on him, as Mussolini promulgated his racial laws in 1938, a clairvoyant Paul—released from the military and serving as a law professor at the University of Padua—had changed course to snatch his wife and young children from the dangers to Jews in Italy.

But the Paul I knew had not succeeded in banishing that mistake about fascism. His civic accomplishments, oh yes, proved his devotion to fairness and opportunity for all. Eloquent—he could be eloquent in his profession, in his Sunday lunch talk, at cocktail parties. But it would take a cadre of soldiers to drive out the ancient, unspoken sadness and shame that inhabited his psyche. Perhaps those unnamed emotions had pushed him to hurry, to be ever busy—through a legal brief on to a new case, off to the next cocktail gathering, then to a meeting, and, finally, to swimming solo and writing a memoir. Paul's language had almost slipped away when he began that writing project, for he had already embarked on his helter-skelter journey into Alzheimer's disease.

"I am in a hurry, you know. To save Venice."

"I will leave you to do it now, Paul," for the work of saving your Venice cannot wait. I closed the book and left for home in the twilight of that rainy November afternoon.

—⁂—

Paul died on December 6, 1997, of a massive heart event. Once again the telephone broke into our life: we found, just as we had found in Seattle, a series of messages as we came in from art-gallery hopping and eating spicy chicken wings in the Central West End. The messages directed John to Barnes Hospital, where Silvia stood firmly in her refusal to allow Paul to have a heart bypass operation. As Paul's medical directives spelled out, there would be no heroic measures. Silvia did not flinch as she insisted on following Paul's desires, nor did John, in spite of the medical staff's efforts to override directives and common sense to provide this Alzheimer's-ridden man with magical heart functions.

Nothing about Paul in the autumn of 1997 had signaled that he was about to die. The nurses said he savored his medication-laced ice cream. He walked the halls of his locked unit, greeting one and all. Italian took over once again as his primary language, so that John received occasional calls from nurses asking what a word meant. Except for his Alzheimer's and its side effects, such as lost glasses and clothing and fantastical remarks about his heroic mission to save Venice, Paul seemed in fine fettle.

As far as I knew, Silvia and John and his siblings had barely discussed what would happen when Paul died. Yet, from long-ago conversations with her father, Luciana understood Paul's desire that the Jewish Kaddish or Prayer for the Dead be recited at his burial in the Jewish Cemetery on the Lido, across the lagoon from Venice. I surmised that Paul's finale would be flamboyant and symbolic but had no idea of what that might entail.

It began on the December Saturday when Paul died. First, Paul had to be ritually washed, wound in a simple cloth, and placed in a plain pine coffin. The mortician invited John to participate. John had burst into hives upon crossing the threshold of the maternity ward when Ellen was born. In spite of his valiant help convincing Paul to shower, there was no possibility that John would assist at the ritual washing of his father.

About the burial, John soon uncovered these facts:

- A body must leave the United States for Italy from a point with an Italian consulate. The consul must seal the coffin with a wax seal at the departure point, in this case, an airport tarmac.
- The wooden coffin must be placed inside an official crate, which only some jets can accommodate in their refrigerated cargo holds.
- At the arrival airport in Italy—and there were only two authorized ones—an Italian medical officer must meet the plane and approve the entrance of the body. Note: Such officers do not normally work on weekends.
- John should accompany the body in order to verify papers and procedures.
- Contrary to the usual Jewish prohibition against embalming, the body has to be preserved for public health reasons.

John and Luciana, who had come to St. Louis to help, telephoned relatives, officials, and clergy in Italy from our dining room table. We ate a crate of tangerines and worked for several days until about 2 p.m. St. Louis time or early evening in Italy. Silvia sat with us but bowed out of logistics. She decided not to go to Italy for the burial. In fact, we weren't sure whether she grasped that Paul had died, so vague and detached was she at this time. Grief itself may have shut Silvia down. Yet with hindsight, we discovered that Silvia's decisive clarity at the hospital fit a pattern of early Alzheimer's disease: an ability to rise to an extraordinary situation. Soon after, she reverted to disengagement.

I stayed at home to plan Paul's St. Louis memorial service and to help Silvia. Albert couldn't leave his job to go to Venice at that time; he and his family came to St. Louis for the memorial.

John and Luciana garnered time dispensations from a rabbi and assurances that a consular official would be present in Chicago and Rome. Luciana had to return to Boston before meeting John in Venice. John waited in St. Louis for tickets for himself and his father's body. But when he and Paul's body arrived in Chicago, logistics went awry. In spite of two reservations on Delta airlines—one for John and one for a coffin—at the last moment, Paul's coffin in its packing crate wouldn't fit in the Delta hold and had to be sent via Alitalia. On the tarmac after the Italian consular official had sealed the crate with an official wax seal, John waved it on its way and boarded his Delta flight.

Venice that December, as John tells the tale, was sparkling clear, the water and sky dancing in the brilliant Mediterranean light. Various kin still active in the Venetian Jewish community stepped forward to offer assistance with the Jewish and Venetian authorities. On the appointed day, John and Luciana and family boarded two municipal funeral boats, confident in having collected enough second cousins' high-school age sons to complete a minyan of ten Jewish men. As the boats were about to sail across to the Lido, Paul's beloved first cousin Giovannina, a statuesque old lady with an aquiline nose, turned to John:

"I am relieved that we have a minyan. I wasn't sure we could arrange one, John."

"Thank you, Giovannina, for your help. Thank you for all of us."

"Your father had a long connection with the Jewish community here. I'm glad you could see it firsthand." Giovannina straightened her shoulders and held the collar of her mink coat snugly around her neck.

John told me afterward how he had felt his father's attachment to Venice and to his extended family. In spite of the difficulties and expenses of transporting their father's body to Italy, he and Luciana had shown their love for Paul and their respect for his family.

The two funeral boats motored out into the Grand Canal past the family homes, past a cousin's palazzo with a garden deck overlooking the Grand Canal. Bouncing, they crossed the luminous, choppy waters of the lagoon out to the Lido.

Paul's coffin was unloaded onto a waiting cart, pulled by a small tractor. John, the oldest male relative, led a procession of male family members, followed by Luciana, cousin Giovannina, and the women. They all wound through the streets of the Lido to the cemetery, through its mossy stone gates to a small chapel. Instructing the men to place their hands on Paul's coffin, the rabbi turned to John.

"Now please offer a blessing for your father. Either Hebrew or Italian will do."

No warning before, no time to think: John told me how amazed he was to find himself uttering words of blessing in Italian for his father. The rabbi read the Kaddish, as Paul had long ago stipulated to Luciana; the body was commended to the earth; the Italian adventurer returned to the resting place of his ancestors beneath cypress trees and moss, where sounds of the sea whisper across the island. I think often of Paul there at peace in Italy, at home next to his mother, whom he never mentioned but whose spirit he surely encountered every day of his life. He was reunited with her and his family, his ancestors, his homeland. His suffering was over. His life had come full circle.

Three days later, John called me from New York; he had flown home via Kennedy airport this time.

"Susan, go look on my dresser."

"Why? Tell me how you are." I was glad to know John was homeward bound after I'd spent a week alone at home. Our old basset hound, Winston, had died in October. Without our dog, without the near-daily nursing home crisis calls about Paul, without John, it was too quiet at our house. Lonesome and anxious about John's well-being, I had listened to a tape of Elvis Presley singing "Peace in the Valley" over and over again.

"I'm in a holding room at the airport."

"What does that mean? You're in the States, aren't you?"

"Yup. Just go see if my passport is on my dresser."

Phone in hand, I began to uncover John's dresser stuff. Sure enough, there was his valid American passport, seven days after his departure for Italy.

"Guess what, Suze, I've done this whole trip—traveling, getting cash, and lots of it for the funeral expenses—I've done it all using Dad's passport."

"Your dad's passport? So they're detaining you in New York?"

"I explained to the immigration people that my father had just died and I'd taken his body to be buried on the Lido. They're letting me come home, Suze."

Peace in the valley some day, pace, pax, shalom, in one of the many tongues we speak in our family.

6

My Self
1998

After Paul's death, Silvia rarely mentioned him. Perhaps she spoke of him with Sharon, whose role as social worker/counselor diminished as Silvia settled into her new residence. The fourth-floor unit with its east-facing balcony offered Silvia abundant space and light for her basil plants, as well as the potted dracaena and rubber tree she had brought from poolside at her house. A guest bedroom and bath made comfortable quarters when Luciana visited with her.

Between Silvia's bedroom and bath lay a dressing room. The shelves spilled sweaters, purses, including her tan nylon travel bags, and vividly colored shawls—fringed, embroidered, sparkling with gilt thread; peasant wool from Sicily, Indian silk shantung, fine Italian paisley. But in the living room, Silvia kept clutter hidden away. John helped her fill the room with elegant, polished fruitwood pieces shipped from Italy after World War II. Straight Victorian chairs with a matching settee served as seating, uncomfortable because they felt as if they were stuffed with horsehair. The galley kitchen offered the necessary conveniences—microwave, refrigerator, stove, and dishwasher—without being inviting. Most residents in this retirement center bought a meal plan for eating either in an old-fashioned dining room with white table linens or in a more casual setting, where book groups, a residents' council, and a current events club also met.

John often picked up Silvia and brought her for Sunday lunch at our house. Occasionally we included my parents. My parents and John's had been friends for decades, not intimates but participants in a monthly discussion group, allies in political campaigns, and fellow supporters of the United Nations Association. When my parents rented a cottage close to ours in Michigan, John's often visited at the same time. The four got along well and doted on our children.

As she aged, my mother became squeamish when faced with friends' frailties and ailments. She would not acknowledge Alzheimer's disease, such as Paul's, as if it were hyperbole or a passing medical fad. If I mentioned Silvia's slowing down, she dismissed it with "Enough said." On those Sundays after Paul died, with the three parents as our guests, I felt myself slipping into a caregiving role. I orchestrated seating, steadied parents as they stood up after an hour at the table, and spoke directly and loudly toward Silvia's good ear. At the same time, I was reminded of how positions had shifted. Mom had offered me motherly tips well into my forties:

"If you dress nicely, you'll feel good about yourself. May I treat you to a new dress this spring?" or "I'd like to offer you a new winter coat. After all, you wear it almost daily." The winter coat offer had come at a time when John and I were paying school tuition for all three of our children. I welcomed generous surprise gifts from my mother for she was attuned to the financial restraints on young families like ours. For her, an attractive, careful appearance signaled a well-tended inner spirit.

Even though Mom and I had seldom done "girl things" together, like clothes shopping or getting our nails done, I remained within her sphere of influence, a disciple of her belief in appearances. In an eye-catching way, she was meticulous about her grooming, clothes, and makeup. And private. I was ever curious.

In my childhood house, Mom's clothes, cosmetics, and artifacts were enclosed in a mysterious closet with built-in cedar cabinets. A long beaded cord just inside the door pulled on the closet light. If I were lucky, I could shut myself in her closet without fear of the dark. Each cabinet opened with a little brass knob that I had to turn to peek at her silky underwear and nylon stockings. She folded her knit dresses in one of the cabinets about the right height for me to open when I was 8 or 9 years old. I loved the colors, a warm red and royal blue, but the knit dresses made me uneasy because I thought they fit my mother too tightly. Her theater makeup and face powder were high up on top: the theater makeup out of my reach; the face powder loose, so that I didn't dare reach for the tortoise shell box for fear that it would spill and, like the trap set for Tristan and Iseult, reveal that I had explored my mother's domain.

That makeup lived in the closet as a memento of my mother's theater days; she had played East Coast summer stock and little theater in St. Louis. In 1931, a Gloucester, Massachusetts, newspaper review of a British play, *Nine Till Six*, said: "The honors of the evening go to Miss Dorothy Coleman for her characterization of Miss Roberts, the millinery saleswoman." The reviewer called my mother's performance "as excellent an amateur characterization as this writer has ever seen."

The summer after her college graduation, her father, my Granddaddy Coleman, permitted Mom to go to the utopian arts colony at Chautauqua, New York, to "do opera."

"I sang in choruses, you know. The Cleveland Orchestra played. Once in awhile they needed a maid as a walk-on. I did that, too."

That's how my mother came to know every word in *Carmen* in French. She had been a walk-on who later hummed for my dad the flamenco-like tunes of an opera probably too risqué for his tastes.

When she moved back to St. Louis after four years at Vassar and a fifth year at the University of Missouri School of Journalism, where she received a second bachelor's degree, she sang and acted around St. Louis, rehearsing and performing at night. During the day she wrote features, advice columns, and society news for the *St. Louis Post-Dispatch*. She referred to herself as a "newspaper gal." Saucy, with dark eyebrows, my mother had a dare-me tilt to her head that reflected her independent streak, manifest in her theater adventures and pursuit of a professional degree in the early 1930s. She celebrated that spirited era of her life with studio portraits of herself, arch as she posed in profile—sometimes with a hat—like the celebrity photos of movie stars.

In her bedroom closet, she kept a tin case of stage makeup—grease paint and kohl. As a child, I was forbidden to touch the case by myself, but one rainy Saturday, my mother drew blue kohl under my eyes and rubbed red grease paint into my cheeks. We stood in front of a long mirror on her closet door so that I could admire my doll-like look. The makeup case, I understood, lived in the closet as an emblem of the past when she was an independent, single woman, an actress in community theater productions.

She didn't completely forsake the theater. Her theater books and play scripts sat on shelves near the fireplace in reach of a rocking chair in her bedroom. Many dated from that life before I was born, before she married Dad. Of some plays, such as Noel Coward's, she owned multiple copies for the Sunday evenings when our parents invited friends to read roles aloud. My brother, sister, and I fended for ourselves in the kitchen after Mom had prepared a fragrant party supper of chicken breasts with white wine and green grapes to serve on her blue-speckled Dedham pottery. The adult voices alternated as they read roles. We three kids ate supper in the kitchen, listening to the hilarity and drama of our parents' play-reading party. Later, the theatrical buzz from downstairs rose up to my third-floor bedroom.

Mom's sense of drama was the core of a self that flowered in the theater and continued in her awareness of how to use her voice and how to present herself. Her dressing ceremony was private and privileged. It produced alluring results, based on laws of fashion that she enunciated and I believed for years such as, "Ladies don't wear orange," or "Turtlenecks aren't ladylike," or "In our family, we never wear leopard print." She still abided by classic fashion principles—taupe shoes and open toed sandals for summer only, black suede pumps for winter, raincoat to match outfit, correct hose color for the clothes and the occasion.

As a young woman, I flaunted some of her notions. For her, high heels with slacks were forbidden. When she saw me after work, dressed in my usual heels and pants suit, she raised her eyebrows as if to say, "So that's what they're wearing now."

During the 1980s, Mom minded my clothing and my appearance, and Dad invited me for an official lunch once or twice a year with an agenda focused on me and on our family's financial welfare. Seated at a lunch table in a dark-gray suit with a striped tie, he looked like a British barrister in the way he held his head and peered over the top of his half-glasses. His full lips, however, revealed a sensuality that contrasted with his tall, commanding demeanor. He checked with me that our family had what he considered appropriate insurance coverage for every contingency—auto and homeowners, disability and life, and health.

On those lunch dates, I felt both protected and proud: protected just as I'd felt as a young girl when he shepherded me onto a trolley for a Saturday ride downtown. We would stop at his law firm, and I'd sit on a slippery leather chair in his office. I swung my feet while he leafed through the Saturday mail stacked on his desk. He took me to lunch at the Stix, Baer and Fuller tearoom. We always finished with a chocolate sundae. I felt small and safe and special.

I also felt proud of my dad when I was in elementary school.

One day, he said, "Chickadee, how would you like to be in a parade?"

"What, how, whose parade?" my words tumbled out pell-mell.

"Around the Flynn Park school yard. In a rented convertible."

Our neighborhood elementary school sat in a small urban park with some berms, a few spring-flowering red bud trees, pine trees for hide-and-seek, and a stand of bushes far enough from the school building so that my girlfriends and I could play princess behind them without the boys taunting us.

"Why, Dad? Why a parade with us?"

"There's always a good reason for a parade. This will be with balloons and maybe a clown. We'll be with my school board friends."

"Me alone with you?" I felt honored.

In that Flynn Park parade year, he was an elected member of our local school board. The idea was for board members and their children to connect with their constituents, be visible at the schools. Convertibles, balloons, hard candies tossed to those who watched—all a late 1940s Dick-and-Jane-like project.

On parade day, Dad and I sat in the car's back seat. Mr. O, the gym teacher, drove the car, festooned with red, white, and blue balloons. Dad stood up, gave his politician's clenched-hands wave, as if to urge on the gathered children, teachers, and a few parents. My school friends lined the sidewalk, clapping with delight at being released from class, and I waved at them. That day, to my 9-year-old eyes, my father was an important person, worthy of starring in a parade.

—◊—

Forty years later at one of our lunches, he ordered a bacon, lettuce, and tomato sandwich, the same as always, for he was a man of enduring, simple tastes.

"Now, Chickadee, I'm not trying to pry. And I don't want John to get the impression that he is not providing well. But if you should ever need anything or get in a jam, I'm here." Dad would look steadily at me to see whether this time I had come to him in financial need. While I felt protected, I also was proud of John's and my independence. I never asked Dad for financial aid.

It took my dad time to accept that John wasn't the sole provider and that I was a professional academic who intended not to "fall back on teaching" but to immerse myself in university life wholeheartedly. Once he acknowledged my profession, I tapped his wisdom about people and organizations for guidance in my academic and community involvement. In turn, I discovered he had an academic side. A believing, practicing Presbyterian, Dad had a wealth of biblical knowledge. He was fascinated by the Dead Sea Scrolls and had put together a thorough program, illustrated by maps and documents, which he presented to interested church and international affairs groups.

At one lunch after our financial routine, he said, "I noticed that a book reviewer used the term 'reliable narrator.' Have you ever heard of that term?"

"We throw it around a lot, Dad. It's pretty useful. In life, even."

"How did you learn about it?"

"It was one of the first critical concepts we studied in grad school, part of what we call 'lit crit.' If you can't believe the story's or novel's narrator, then the reader has to work really hard."

"I'll have to think about that. Have you considered the idea with Conrad, say?" Conrad and Kipling were his favorite writers.

"Dad, I teach French literature. I haven't looked at Conrad since high school."

"Well then, could I read something in English that you work on so we could talk about it?" He paused. "Translation must create a whole layer of confusion. And I never could do French. It's an embarrassing language to try to speak with those silly sounds."

Thanks to his curiosity, the reliable narrator entered his life. So did T'ai Chi, which I was learning. He asked me to demonstrate and pronounced the movements "very graceful." Learning began to flow from me to him.

But lunches with my father slowly disappeared, as did Mom's snippets of concerned advice over the years. My father's focus, like Silvia's and Mom's, centered on his own, ever-narrower world.

—⁕—

That summer of 1998, Silvia reveled in the warm sunshine during one Sunday lunch at our house, outside in the shade of our large crabapple tree. After espresso, she tilted her head back with closed eyes. The deep lines on her face softened in the afternoon light. At that time, John and I overlooked many warning signs: Silvia became forgetful, less able to organize herself, confused about day or time, and fearful that her silver would be stolen—in combination, indicators that Alzheimer's disease was taking hold.

Opening her eyes, Silvia said, "I enjoy those grasses." She nodded at a stand of decorative grass that John had planted, "And the way they move in the breeze."

She pointed at John's fern and hosta garden in the shade of our house:

"How did you learn to garden so well?"

"Mamma, from you," he answered. Those three words captured all his devotion to his mother.

Smiling with pleasure, Silvia dozed again.

In June, John received a call from an old man who lived in Silvia's apartment complex. He asked if he might invite Silvia out for dinner. First, however, he asked two questions:

"John, may I ask, is your mother still compos mentis?"

"She's quite something, " I heard John answer.

"Now, more delicately, is she still continent?"

I overheard John chuckle assurances; the gentleman phoned Silvia. She demurred, saying that she needed her son's permission. When she telephoned, John reminded his mother that she was not required to consult him about her social life. But before a "date" could happen, the old fellow shifted his new Buick convertible into reverse in a supermarket parking lot, hit the accelerator instead of the brakes, smashed several cars, and broke his hip. He never followed up on his invitation. Silvia's life narrowed to outings with us and with Pat, who continued to be her full-time housekeeper, aide, and companion.

That same summer, my 89-year-old father lost weight. Mom became a tired, yet stubborn caregiver, trying to tempt Dad to eat high-calorie foods like ice cream. She clung to a life that was hard to maintain in their old age: a big white frame house with nearly two acres of lawn, trees, flower beds, and a tennis court; social and civic activities, such as monthly discussion group dinners, board meetings of Planned Parenthood for Mom and church elders' meetings for Dad; standing lunch dates with friends; and a university course to expand their horizons. The only aspect of their lives they had relinquished by this time was travel, which had become too daunting to plan and too exhausting to carry through.

In the summer, they preserved mealtime ceremonies, even though Mom knew little about cooking and found kitchen cleanup distasteful. She hadn't handled meal preparation for decades because until just a few years before, she and Dad had employed a full-time cook and housekeeper named Dorothy Cross. Dorth came to work for our family when Missy was born and stayed nearly fifty years. She was chocolate-milk brown, sturdy, and straight as an arrow in her posture and moral code. She rolled her hair at night so that each day her hair lay in glossy waves. Dorth's face seemed bemused and calm, her features spreading wide with frequent, warm smiles. Every day she wore a green or yellow uniform with snaps down the front and an apron to match. On dinner party nights when she cooked and stayed late to serve and clean up, Dorth wore a dressy black uniform and a white starched apron, both with lace trim. On those party nights, I sat on the green enamel stool in the kitchen to watch her knead the dough for rolls. Her hands were strong, their palms a wondrous pink brown.

Dorth and Mom were like two facets of the same person. Two Dorothys almost the same age, though born under different signs of the zodiac: Mom, an emotional and dramatic Pisces, and Dorth, a nurturing, motherly Cancer. We called Dorothy the cook Dorth; friends called my mother Dottie. Mom could out-organize and out-manage most CEOs with her keen eye for detail and concomitant sense of the big picture, evident in her leadership on women's issues, particularly reproductive and abortion rights. Dorth could do the same on the domestic front. For Dorth, indeed, managed the day-to-day operations of our household. She was wise and even-tempered as she cared for us three children. When my younger brother, George, tangled with a neighborhood bully who trapped him in an old wooden barrel, Dorth stepped into the fray, rescued George, and sent the bully packing. At the kitchen table, she meted out harsh words for me when I was bossy with my siblings or the neighbor kids. She hugged me when I came crying to her after a neighborhood fracas. Her standards were high, and her heart was big.

Devotion to the well-being of our family bound my mother and Dorth. Dorth allowed Mom the freedom to develop a public presence, while Mom gave Dorth domestic responsibility along with Social Security, vacations, and the green, yellow, and black uniforms Mom insisted she wear. There were occasional tensions between the two women, probably when Dorth asserted herself too much. But we three children and Dad wouldn't tolerate a word of criticism from Mom about Dorth because we all adored and depended on her.

Dorth owned the kitchen and the laundry room in the basement. I shadowed her. I perched on a stool to watch her iron Dad's shirts. From Dorth, I learned how to do a cuff and a collar by watching her angle the hot iron—fragrant in its steamy smell—so that it smoothed the collar points with never a wrinkle, never the need for a second pass. I sat in the kitchen as she rolled up cinnamon buns or snapped green beans or stood back from the stove to keep the fried chicken from splattering her apron. She sang hymns from her church, where she was an usher, and reminded me of what the Bible said when I needed scolding—things about obeying your parents and behaving, which usually meant not racing bikes with the neighborhood boys. She lavished affection on her nieces and on us. The widow of a railroad conductor, Dorth had no children of her own.

One day after nearly a half century at our house, Dorth arrived at work and asked Mom for a raise. The story I heard came from Dad, who'd heard it from Mom:

"Mrs. R., I believe that I am due for a raise about now. It has been quite awhile."

"Dorothy Cross," there was surely an edge in my mother's voice as she addressed Dorth with her full name, "Raises aren't something that a person is due."

"I've been working for you for more than forty years. I have had some raises. I believe I'm due for another one now."

"You notice that your hours have become shorter, Dorothy. True, there are just my husband and me, and there is less to do. Less to do. Fewer hours. So the same pay covers fewer hours, which is the equivalent of a raise."

"Well, Mrs. R., I'm an old lady like you. I'm thinking ahead. It's a long drive out here. I need a raise."

"I am sorry, but I cannot give you a raise."

"Then this will be my last day of work."

I imagine that with her usual goodwill and sense of responsibility, Dorth composed herself and went about the morning routine. She washed the breakfast dishes, made my parents' bed, emptied the wastebaskets and stacked up the old newspapers, set the table for lunch, and chopped apples and walnuts for a Waldorf salad. From the tiny first-floor bathroom, she collected the baggy gray sweater she kept for chilly days, her comb, the hose she wore with her dress uniform, and a bottle of hand lotion. She left after just a few hours; neither she nor my mother said goodbye.

Dad called to tell me that Dorth no longer worked for them. I hoped he was outraged that these two potent women had parted company stubbornly and abruptly. Missy was upset because Dorth had been at home for her when Mom began work—first, at the St. Louis Art Museum doing publicity, then teaching high school English part-time. George and I were saddened, cautious about the consequences of this rupture. We all kept in touch with Dorth through Christmas gift exchanges and occasional requests for a batch of cinnamon rolls, which gave us a chance to visit with her. When Dorth died four years after she and Mom parted company, Dad, Mom, Missy, and I attended the visitation at a St. Louis funeral home. In the car we shared tales of Dorth humming as she baked her legendary burnt sugar cake in her kitchen kingdom.

Dorth's departure ushered in a new era. Mom became the household cook, and a cleaning service whizzed through the house every other week. Preserving the graceful routines of mealtime proved daunting for Mom, who had cooked very little. As Dad aged, his appetite diminished while his puritanical relationship to food grew more marked. He expected plain food to sustain him along with plenty of sweets, yet he believed that kitchen or food work was beneath the women in our family. One summer when our daughter Carol found a job as a hostess at a pasta restaurant, Dad pulled me aside:

"Is Carol really going to work in a restaurant?"

"Yep," I said, chuckling to myself, knowing this would be a dad inquisition.

"What kind of place is it?"

"Spaghetti and stuff, Dad." He never caught on to the notion of "pasta."

"Well, I have a proposition for you."

"Okay, Dad, let's hear it."

"I don't want our family in the food business. How about if I pay her what she could earn there, and then she could enjoy her summer at a camp or something."

"No, Dad. She got this job herself. It'll be an important experience."

In France in 1959–60, during my junior year in college, I learned that I loved to cook and to eat. Both of my parents accused me of having become "sybaritic" during that year in Paris. It was an odd choice of

word, but whenever Mom or Dad called me "sybaritic," it was a criticism. Once I angered them right after I came back from Paris by asking
for freshly ground pepper and questioning why our family didn't own a
pepper mill. I was a condescending 21-year-old, certain after Paris that
life in the Midwest with stodgy parents and no pepper mill was a thing
of my past. I also had enough of a contrary streak to want to embrace a
culinary life distinct from my parents' world of fried chicken, angel food
cake, and Dorth's all-day green beans.

But sybaritic wasn't the right word, nor was it what I became in
France. That word reflected Dad's attitude toward food lovers, which
might explain why he was so thin throughout his life. Eating—except
bacon, lettuce, and tomato sandwiches, chocolate sundaes, and broken
milk-chocolate chunks—was a necessary evil. Mom harbored her own
mother's love of folksy fare, such as sweet rolls and Dorth's burnt sugar
cake. Mom ate heartily but often skipped salads, crisp vegetables ("which
you young people like"), and fresh fruit. Even though she pretended to
scorn highfalutin cuisine, she savored fancy dishes of lobster and soufflés
in restaurants.

I loved my time in the kitchen: I read recipes, chopped and minced,
tasted and tested seasoning, beat and sliced. I taught myself all these
techniques from Julia Child's first French cookbook. One evening my
friend Lillian phoned at dinner time.

"What are you making tonight?"

"I have a couple of cookbooks out," I said. "I've got some cream and
some mushrooms and a chicken. I don't know yet."

"Aren't you tired from work?"

"It's how I relax," I answered. "It's a whole other world. None of the
same brain cells. No student crises to solve."

Then I added, "You know, cooking and meals are holy to me. Like a sacrament."

Admittedly, it was hard to find dinner preparation sacred with three young children circling around, asking when we were going to eat and whether they could watch one more TV show, while two dogs played underfoot. John usually came home late, as he pushed himself in his law practice. I would tackle a stack of French essays once the kids were in bed. Equally difficult was picturing dinner time as holy a few years later, when our three high school kids slouched in late from sports, dropping hockey sticks and a football helmet on the floor. Will gulped down a quart of milk, and each one reminded me of food restrictions—no salt, I hate red meat, don't give me tomatoes, I'm becoming a vegetarian, and I'm not eating because I have too much homework. I held steady with the dinner routine even though I was mad at teenage strictures and stymied by adolescent moods. Over dinner, night after night, we connected for thirty minutes as a family, linked by shared tales and pastas and endless variations on ground beef and complaints about stupid teachers. For a special occasion, I might try my version of a fragrant stew that simmered while I read at home to prepare the next day's class.

Family dinners, like Sunday lunches, knit us together, unless: unless one child threw a "tizzy fit" or one teased another or the phone rang incessantly or another child had only 10 minutes to eat. Or John grumped about a shortage of grated cheese. Or I was too tired to notice that we were, indeed, knitted together like the stitches in a sweater, the first stitch holding the next, which holds the next, and so on.

—⁓—

Born in that year of mine in Paris—maybe when I took myself alone to a bistro at three o'clock in the afternoon, where I ordered a dozen snails, red wine, plenty of bread, and then wallowed in the garlicky parsley butter sauce—born that day were my willingness to taste foods and my desire to replicate and invent my own dishes. After that Parisian year, eating solo was replaced by a growing sense of meals as both ceremonial and communal.

By the time my mother took on meal preparation in the mid-1990s, she and I had made our peace about cuisine. I had transformed the language and literature skills developed during my year in France into a doctorate and then a university position teaching French; cooking became one of my pastimes. Mom, in her post-Dorth years, asked me for advice and recipes, as she tackled dishes like chocolate mousse. She bought herself a coffee bean grinder and an enameled cast-iron casserole. After dinner, Dad rolled up his sleeves and loaded dishes into the dishwasher. The cooking and cleanup framed their lifelong habit of cocktails first, then dinner in the dining room in winter or on the screen porch in summer, and dessert, which usually included ice cream. Yet, keeping up the old ways became a strain on my mother. She complained that she didn't have enough ideas for meals and wasn't comfortable leaving Dad alone while she grocery shopped. Mom left house cleaning to the service, didn't own a vacuum, and contented herself with tidying, so that her house always looked presentable. Not that she was afraid of hard work. She knew how to lobby the Missouri legislature on behalf of women's reproductive rights. Like a play producer, she could organize and chair a meeting—she was an expert at such public undertakings. But she was becoming worn down by planning and fixing meals, and Dad was getting feeble and demanding.

In the summer of 1998, Dad fell several times, lost a hearing aid, but was cheerful throughout. Mom was tired and miserable after having a root canal procedure. I sensed my mother's tension about life in their big house and wondered whether my parents needed more help. She and my dad could no longer organize themselves to travel, not even to Lake Michigan, where there were too many steps inside the house and over the dunes down to the beach for either one to tackle. While we were in Pentwater, I tried not to hash over my parents' future with John as we took long walks on the beach. I promised myself to face the situation after the vacation. John and I played tennis and enjoyed time with Will and his fiancée, Sara. They had become engaged in the spring. The four of us looked ahead to the wedding.

I felt like a creature with two selves, two I's—the eleven-months-of-the-year self and the July-in-Pentwater self. My July self was relaxed and tolerant, a respite from my usual oldest-child, driven self. Proust's narrator speaks about having many "I's," multiple *moi*. Sometimes there seem to be so many Proustian selves that parsing them challenges the most accomplished, perceptive critics. I was a far simpler character than Proust's narrator, an eleven-months self and a July one.

Each March when I received a note from the owner of the cottage we had rented for more than thirty years, the prospect of July in Michigan was as welcome as the spring equinox. With her note, my horizons opened onto a pine and birch forest. In my mind's eye, I saw the dunes that rolled down from the cottage to Lake Michigan, whose waves sounded in my ears as I wrote a deposit check and a return note, ushering in the first sensations of my July self.

July started after we traversed Illinois cornfields, turned north at Effingham, battled traffic around Chicago, then broke into the first sandy dunes of Indiana, which presaged our Michigan dunes. When we turned into the densely wooded driveway in Pentwater, I was breathless. Nothing was as dark as those towering woods, nothing as bright as the sun filtering through onto the forest floor. Shafts of light moved across dead oak leaves, myriad mosses, and fallen rotting trees. The canopy of trees thinned as the expanse of Lake Michigan surged into view. We opened the car's windows, breathed in pine-fragrant air, ready for the arrival moment, ready for linkage to past moments.

Nana Coleman, my mother's mother, traveled to Pentwater in 1916 with her two oldest children, Dorothy and Mamie. Granddaddy Coleman had scouted a place far removed from the unhealthy St. Louis heat and humidity. He sent his family north on the train with steamer trunks, Mom told me. Although she only spent a few summers in Pentwater as a child, it entered her subconscious. Soon after World War II, she and Dad began renting cottages right on Lake Michigan in Pentwater. So my own Julys took shape—water and sand, dunes and woods—an immense playground for Missy, George, and me, with my last childhood summer there in 1959, as I prepared to go to France for my junior year of college. I was frightened of the year's adventure ahead of me, rude to my parents, and domineering with Missy, who was 12. I lay in the dunes, isolated from everyone and reading Joyce's *Ulysses*, for which Mom signed a library permission slip because legally I was too young for such material.

Those dunes and that immense lake had cradled me as I grew into adulthood. I had to offer this same chance to my own children. I wanted John to share this part of myself, born in Julys so long ago. I wanted my family to understand that here lay the fundamental joys of my life. Here, too, the peaceful, steady, loving July self was my favorite self, the one I aspired to all year long.

For more than thirty years, Pentwater had allowed John and me to read aloud or barbecue or walk miles on the beach, roaming over our lives or accepting our silence. At times, that Michigan nourishment of our relationship buoyed us during the other eleven months of the year, especially during the demanding periods of professional development and child rearing.

In Pentwater, John loved to buy a stack of the day's newspapers— the *Wall Street Journal*, the *Detroit Free Press*, and the *New York Times*.

He sprawled on our bed wearing next to nothing, sheets thrown back, windows and door open onto the balcony that looked west over Lake Michigan. The afternoon wind billowed the blue-striped curtains, voices rose from the beach below, and sunlight bathed the room. Downstairs on the porch, I stretched on an old wicker chaise longue, reading a big novel, such as *Gone with the Wind*.

John called down, "Suze, what are you doing down there on the porch?"

Minutes later the next call: "Suze, how about a nap?"

Now that we often were alone in the cottage, John scarcely needed his euphemistic invitation from our child-rearing years: "Suze, why don't you come up and play?" The third call harked back to the codes we hoped our children didn't understand. With all the cottage doors and windows open to the summer breeze and sunshine, we embraced each other and the mid-July afternoon.

I loved, too, the bits of family conversation echoing through the cottage from our children's past—icons of their development, markers of the passage of time, distilled once a year into that twelfth month of July. For that was what our days in Michigan were—a distillation of where we had been and how we had evolved over the past year.

I recalled Ellen, our oldest child, at about age 9, writing and directing plays with her brother and sister and their friends, as she put every detail in order, down to hand-lettered programs and popcorn sales. Often she cast herself as the queen, who reigned from the wicker chaise longue wearing a glittery aluminum foil crown. One July Will lay on the back deck, lifting weights to build muscles for football. Etched forever was the image of our younger daughter Carol at age 22, setting off in a used car for two months alone in the national parks. Fresh from her college graduation, with her beautiful curly hair, confident in her coping and camping skills, Carol disappeared through the shelter of our woods onto a highway going west. I waved, then cried, as I kicked sand along the path back to the cottage.

All the generations figured in my memories: beach parties where a 4-year-old's voice sang as loudly as an 80-year-old's. I thought of Missy and her family, George, Mom and Dad, John, our children and multitudes of their friends, and Paul and Silvia during numerous summers. The stories of my grandmother, aunts and uncles, and many cousins washed over me.

There were also ferocious moments in Pentwater. Slashing thunderstorms roared across the lake as jags of lightning sliced a black sky and thunder shook the old cottage's frame. Trees bent to slap the windows. Lights flickered and went off. Horizontal sheets of rain raced over the lake, hitting the cottage like knives. Storms in my own life, storms in our family's life banged our foundations: easy-to-weather storms like emergency trips to nearby Ludington Hospital for Ellen's appendectomy and Dad's knee, broken while playing family doubles tennis, or St. Louis crises muted as we listened to them over the phone. Fierce storms with our children or our parents had smashed the summer calm, battered some Julys. These upheavals left dangerous broken trees and downed wires in their wake. But, like the storms off the lake, the most fearsome family storms slowly blew away, bringing again the brilliance of July days.

In 1998, John and I played tennis, walked on the beach, swam, read, chatted. We each had private time—I on a boardwalk bench with a 180-degree panorama of Lake Michigan, John on rambles in search of freshly picked local raspberries. Those times let us settle inside ourselves and explore how next to deal with our parents. We floated our doubts and anxieties, testing approaches to our eleven-month lives. I mapped a fall syllabus for intermediate French; caught up on professional literature about second language acquisition; laughed at best sellers, like Rebecca Wells's *Divine Secrets of the Ya-Ya Sisterhood*; and admired serious books, such as Bernhard Schlink's *The Reader*. I went home to St. Louis rested, peaceful, hopeful that the other three parents' declines would not be as turbulent as Paul's.

In August 1998, my father fell again. He had begun a season of falls in the previous winter that made him stiff until spring. When he fell in August, Dad's travel files could have killed him. He kept the files in an old steel cabinet at the bottom of the basement stairs. Dad categorized trips alphabetically, with rust red manila envelopes for the material from major travels and thin white files for minor trips, labeled with destination and date. The files began with Afghanistan—that trip was in 1974. The trips marched across the world, sometimes with two visits to one place, such as India or Balbianello on Lake Como in Italy. There was a file for East Africa and one for South Africa. Dad was in his eighties for that trip, an organized tour. He took time from group outings to visit fellow Presbyterians in Cape Town. On this tour, Dad and Mom also viewed game from a Land Rover in Botswana and Zimbabwe. In a letter to our family from his final African trip, Dad spoke of seeing "lots of wart hogs running with their silly tails straight up like flags, hyenas, a cheetah with cubs . . . and in spite of searching hard we saw no leopard—our only miss among the animals." He and Mom visited Russia when it was still the Soviet Union, traveled to Turkey, Scotland and the Hebrides. They drove the length of a medieval pilgrimage route in northern Spain. There were no files for Southeast Asia or Japan. I guessed that Dad had no desire to return to that part of the world after his posting to the Pacific in World War II.

That August day at home, Dad stumbled and fell near the bottom of the stairs. He grabbed the top file drawer handle. The fully loaded cabinet rocked forward onto its front corners. In the split second before he involuntarily released his grip, the cabinet balanced forward and threatened to tip over onto him. But the 5-foot-tall cabinet did not fall. The weight of those files, spanning years and coursing the globe, didn't crush my father as they might have. In an anthropomorphic way, in a grace-filled moment, the cabinet's bulk of steel and heavy paper refused to take my father's life. Instead, Dad fell directly in front of it, where he lay crumpled on the floor for a minute, as he told the tale, then pushed himself up and found the file he wanted.

Dad's advanced medical directives instructed Mom, Missy, George, and me—yes, "instructed" us because that was how Dad talked about end-of-life matters—that no one should do anything extraordinary to prolong his life. Tubes and feeding lines, heroic resuscitation, and respirators were all rejected in his legal documents. He would be in charge of his dying, for he was accustomed to controlling his and his clients' issues of life and death: finances, wills, investments, burial plans, and plots. He could not have predicted that a flaking gray cabinet would flash a will of its own, spare him, and leave him crumpled on the cool basement floor with only a scraped elbow. Dad was a little bit hurt, flustered by not landing on his feet and not being completely in charge. He had flirted with death, and death refused him the privilege.

After Dad fell a second time in August, I called Missy to register my concerns.

"Hey, Miss, how's it going?"

"What's up?" We both knew from years of habit that these openers signaled "business," not just an idle chat.

"Dad fell again today."

"He did?"

"Yep. It's the third or fourth time in the last few months. He's okay, but I'm really worried."

"About what?"

"About his falling. And how dangerous it is."

"I think you're over-involved in Mom and Dad's life," she said slowly, like a parent explaining to a child. "You take every little thing as a call for you to 'do something.'"

"I'm concerned, really concerned. Wondering whether we should or could do anything."

"You ought to look into yourself. At your motives." My sister's tone seemed flat and clipped. "You ought to ask yourself why you want to get in the middle."

"Well, I do look into myself. It's about love. I worry about the causes and consequences of Dad's falls. He's just been lucky." My answer sounded feeble and defensive, even though I felt hot with anger at my sister. Obviously, my motives were complex. I couldn't possibly sort through them. I didn't want to spend time in self-analysis. Especially not when fall semester was in full swing with new graduate students and freshmen undergraduates. Dad and Mom were my beloved, complicated, aging, strong, dignified, breaking-down, devoted, stoic, failing, needy, independent parents.

"Theirs is just normal old people stuff. You ought to back off and examine yourself, like I said before."

"I hear you." I was stung when Missy chastised me. I was sad, too, at being alone with a sense of duty about Dad's well-being. I wished I were back on the beach in Michigan.

"Are we on for Saturday tennis?" Missy asked. Her voice returned to its easy, natural inflection.

"We're on. I'm ready to hit some balls. Hard. I'll pick you up at two, okay?"

—⁂—

Dad was also losing his capacity to deal with and recall numbers; a doctor called it "innumeracy." The definition of innumerate is "without a basic knowledge of mathematics or arithmetic." Though Dad had studied math and had been an excellent manager of his and others' finances, he could no longer recognize numbers, couldn't add or subtract. Fear of having "lost his fortune"—that old Depression specter of being jobless, which had haunted him from the days after law school when he knocked on law firm doors—drove him to call the family bank trust officer several times a day to check on how much money he had. My mother reported this on the phone, frustrated and embarrassed at my father's unbridled persistence.

"Chickadee," my dad said to me one day, "do you see this slip of paper?" He pulled a tiny crumpled note from his pocket. I looked at it.

"Lots of numbers there, Dad."

"The bank gave them to me this morning. What do they mean? I couldn't figure where to put the point. You know that point? The bank told me there was a point."

The numbers on the slip of paper were 1-2-5-4-9-0-8.

"What did the bank say this was?"

"My money. Do you think I'm a millionaire?"

"I don't know, Dad. I hope so, after all your hard work."

"Would you put the point in? And the dollar sign? And tell me how much I have."

"Okay." I read deliberately, "Twelve thousand five hundred forty-nine dollars and eight cents."

"Is that enough?"

"It's just fine. Plenty for anything."

Dad stood straight and tall that autumn. He'd lost numbers but was temporarily free from falling. A genie, hidden in the Pamir Mountains file or in the record of the Finis Terra rock outcropping off Scotland's Orkney Islands, had held the heavy cabinet upright. My father was still standing. Dad was not, I tried to convince myself, surely was not failing. Mom claimed her cooking was going better. I, like my mother, was keeping up appearances.

7

Managerial Stress
1999

M om lay on the emergency room hospital bed, draped in a white gown with a small blue-dash print like Morse code. The head of the bed was cranked up, bending her at the middle.

When Dad left the room to look for a drinking fountain, Mom said, "I can't do it. I can't manage."

"It's a tough time, Mom." As I listened to my weak reply, I felt ashamed that I didn't have the energy to give my mother more sympathy.

"It's all too much—your father, the house, the meals. And your father couldn't even remember the most basic things he needed today—his driver's license and my insurance cards."

I leaned in toward her on the bed: "What happened to your breast, anyway?" That morning Mom had telephoned to tell me that Dad would drive her the 15 miles to the hospital emergency room used by her doctor. It was about her breast—tenderness, a bruise, and her overarching fears of cancer and being laid low when she was needed as a caregiver. Rather than try to decipher her problem, I agreed to meet them at the emergency room.

"It's nothing." She stopped. "I'm afraid it's breast cancer."

"It looks like only a bruise, Mom." Bruise equals cancer: I acknowledged my mom's fear about how she would manage, her sense of drama, her low pain threshold, and her tendency to grab my father's attention with ailments. I thought, too, of the ungraded French literature papers I'd left on my desk to join my parents at the hospital. Quickly, I pulled myself back to concentrate on Mom, feeling delinquent because my professional obligations were distracting me.

"What would happen to your father if I have breast cancer?"

"Mom, don't jump ahead. A bruise isn't cancer. How'd you get it?"

"Bumping into the bathroom door in the middle of the night." Her head rested back on the bed, making her look far away. "I never go out any more. We never go out. The house is too big. I needed someone to check my breast."

"Someone will be here soon. I'll wait and go back to work after I talk to the doctor."

"I never meant to be a burden. Your father and I tried to organize everything so we wouldn't be a burden on you children." Her voice trailed off as if she wanted to be sure I understood her despair. I did.

"I know, Mom. You aren't a burden. Get some rest. I brought a book to read. I'm prepping for tomorrow, okay?"

"I will if you crank me down. And help me figure out how to manage." Her voice faded as she dozed.

About ten years earlier, I should have suspected that management woes would figure in Mom's aging. Mom coined a phrase at that time when she was still going full tilt: she named her occasional attacks of anxiety "managerial stress."

One day—it seemed eons ago, yet Mom had been in her late seventies—when she was fresh in from playing tennis and had been spending most of her time leading a capital fund drive for a reproductive health cause, she telephoned me as our three children were about to begin summer vacation from college.

"I've got a problem," Mom said. This was not her usual approach.

I asked her what it was.

"Managerial stress," she answered.

Managerial stress, managerial stress, managerial. . . . This term from our conversation years ago resonated in the emergency room as I watched Mom cling to shreds of her management prowess. She had been such a gifted manager—decisive, lucid, smart—wham, bang. She would say, "Let's write the Catholic Church a letter and go see them about opening an abortion dialogue, sit down and talk, be reasonable. Don't say it can't be done. I'll check my calendar for a date. And Dorth, I've written out today's tasks, the menus for meals; you'll see what needs cooking." Mom could have been a leader of industry, the CEO of a large corporation, or a successful theater producer. The play script, the blocking notes, the movements on stage—my mother had also produced them for her volunteer "projects," just as she'd done when she played summer stock in her college years and participated in community theater in St. Louis after college.

As we waited in the emergency room, I thought of how I hadn't wanted her to manage me in the 1980s. I was coming into my own as a manager, as I took responsibility for segments of the French curriculum in my university department and as I balanced the diverse elements of my life. As she had always commented on my appearance, Mom began to keep an eye on my management skills, especially vis-à-vis our increasingly independent children. Knowing her gifts, I could not be resentful, only bemused. Perhaps back in the 1980s, she was exhibiting her first fears of not knowing where and what was going on around her, fears that plagued her now in the spring of 1999. Information—geographical, chronological, strategic—made her feel included in family affairs, if not in control.

"What exactly are your children's summer plans?" she had asked in the early summer of 1989.

Like an auctioneer barking, I called out bits of data as quickly as I could to assuage my mother's management fears—taking tiny breaths, not giving her a chance to cut in:

"Ellen has a job right here in St. Louis, Mom, where she goes every day from 8 to 5 except on Wednesdays when singles meet in the park for beer; yes, she's over 21. Sometimes on Tuesdays and Thursdays she goes to aerobics—you following me, Mom? She loves her job, but she might move back to college with her boyfriend who works in the food business." I tried that instead of saying her boyfriend was working that summer as a "waiter" to avoid my parents' disdain.

Mom had asked if there were anything she could do to help me.

Toward the end of June in 1989, Mom called again. I asked how she was handling her managerial stress.

"I'm wondering," she said, "if you could tell me where each one of your children is at this very moment?" She liked to tease me on occasion. I coughed into the phone.

"Touchée; you got me!" We laughed together. Back then, she had been fun to josh with. Now she was fragile and unsure, navigating the seas of old age. These ten years later, I wondered whether managerial stress was hereditary and would attack me when my own arenas of control shrank. My own old age was too scary to contemplate.

Even though Mom's visible problem that day in the ER was only a bruise, she had told me what was really wrong: she felt overwhelmed and unhappy. She derived no pleasure from cooking and keeping the house.

She and Dad weren't having any fun. The trip to the emergency room was a cry for help. Shortly after this episode, Mom and I hired Judy to be their new housekeeper.

I found it hard to keep our parents' declines in perspective. I caught glimpses of the managerial mountains ahead, especially when I thought about how independent Dad and Mom had been until about a year and a half before. Their future had seemed like a distant, misty landscape in a Dutch genre painting, where you peer into the background for tiny personages—a peasant leading a goat, a couple arm in arm, a plump woman suckling a baby—in hopes that a miniature indication of life afar will augment the painting's foreground story and reveal what lies ahead. As I peered beyond Dad and Mom's daily events, I looked for a passable road in the distance, not a road that dissolved into dark, cracked pigment with no clues as to where it led. Missy, George, and I had not planned for our roles when it became our turn to journey past the familiar, animated foreground of our parents' existence to peer at the picture's far edge, where shapes and paths and boundaries blurred.

On the way to our Saturday tennis game, I told Missy about Mom's bruised breast and her anguish about managing their lives as octogenarians.

"Yeah, and my job sucks, too," she said, driving fast on the highway. "I have a totally stupid employee—she wastes my time with her problems and incompetence."

"Mom and Dad worry me. Not to mention Silvia."

"And my kids, oh god, my kids. . . ." Missy was worried about her children at that time; we could complain to each other as much as we needed to on the way to tennis, sort of a sisterly catharsis.

"Fun and games with our kids and the octogenarians," I said.

"Right now, my woes register about a nine on a ten-point scale, I'd say." Missy's tone was tart.

"Seinfeld could make an episode," I said.

"Or, we could invent a woe-mometer to measure our troubles—all my troubles, Lord," she sang the gospel song's refrain.

"For every problem, you squeeze the woe-mometer and see how high it registers. So, how do we measure?" I asked, squeezing the air in the car with my fist. "Damn big house Mom and Dad live in."

"Thinking about them in that house with all those slippery floors and ancient plumbing—that'll raise the woe level. We could build a woe-mometer and fill it with some kind of liquid to make it look like a giant thermometer. Come on up, folks—a squeeze per woe to see how high you can make our woe-mometer go," said Missy.

"It could be like the hammer swing at a state fair or the blood pressure machine at the super market. Watch to see how high it goes. Give me another ER visit with Mom, and I'll top it at ten."

At the tennis court, my sister said, "Let's play." She popped open a can of new tennis balls. "They'll be okay—Mom and Dad. They've just got the 'usual' for old folks."

"Emergency rooms and breast bruises and falls aren't my idea of the usual. Let's warm up at the net."

"Just hit soft balls. Easy, Susan. You're too much in the middle with Mom and Dad."

—⁂—

Twice within two days in May, Dad had bowel explosions: once with Mom at home and once when Mom was out and Judy, their new housekeeper, was at home with Dad. Mom and I had hired Judy to work 30 hours per week as a housekeeper/caregiver at the beginning of 1999, four or five years after Dorth left. Petite, bustling in the ballet slippers she wore as she worked, Judy called herself a professional housekeeper on her mauve business cards. The kitchen became her domain, as it had been Dorth's. She listened to Mozart, read her daily Bible lesson, and baked. She specialized in baking because, as she reminded me on most of my visits, she had studied with a renowned pastry chef. Her pastries and sweets were delectable and decorated as if by an artist.

With my father, she patiently searched for a letter he had lost or the cash he had withdrawn from the bank. Mom didn't want to cozy up to Judy for fear Judy would try to convert her to join the Jehovah's Witnesses. My mother loved the liturgy and ceremony of her Episcopalian faith. She was not open to exploration of another denomination. From my point of view, Judy brought another perspective to goings-on at Mom and Dad's house. As Dad's bodily functions engulfed the household's life, none of us, including the doctor, could figure out the cause of his bowel problems. His doctors suggested damage to sphincter muscles during radiation treatment for prostate cancer a decade earlier. What had been a "cure" was raising its head in what seemed an ignominious display of bodily control gone haywire. My father complied with food restrictions and medications. Mom ruefully told me that the two of them had studied their medical manuals for a solution to his incontinence, and Dad asked me for a copy of Sherman Nuland's book, *How We Die*. Mom read material to get ideas for relaxation or exercise for her and Dad. Neither one exercised much. They had installed an electric stair lift after Mom's double knee replacement operation in 1994. The surgery did not cure her arthritic pain, leaving climbing the stairs as difficult as before surgery. Nor did my parents stroll down their driveway and along their lane any more. They stopped walking the perimeter of their property to survey the trees my father cherished—a plum planted in honor of a birthday, a giant blue spruce rare in our area, myriad sweet gum trees shading the house. Both used canes on cold, damp days.

In 1999, Dad decided not to drive any longer after he got lost on several outings to familiar places. Judy drove him to the bank frequently to get "cash for the weekend" or to have his account balanced, even though he couldn't decipher the numbers given to him. Several times a month, he lunched with a group of men who called themselves the Peripatetics because they ate at a different place each time. Most of the men were so old that they walked bent over canes or walkers and no longer drove. Mercifully, Ben W.'s chauffeur began the rounds to pick up the men at about 11 a.m. Dad waited at the door, cane ready, tie carefully knotted, a recent *New Yorker* article in mind for discussion, if he could remember its topic by the time they arrived for lunch.

While Dad was having lunch with his friends in the spring of 1999, Mom telephoned me at home. I was preparing a French quiz on my computer.

"I need your father to go out more, to give me some breathing room."

"I hear you, Mom. Are you getting out at all yourself?" I asked.

"Never. It feels like never. I don't have any outings of my own. It's awful."

She sounded distant and flat. Despair laced her words.

"What about your Friday reading group?" I said. "Aren't any of them around?"

The reading group of six or seven of my mother's closest friends had met for more than twenty years on Fridays for sherry, a bring-your-own-sandwich lunch, and a "read." That had meant taking turns reading aloud a biography of Truman, for example. In recent years, the reading tapered off. Kate was legally blind. Maria had a Chilean accent the women found hard to understand, and Patricia had gone deaf. Either Mom or Betty T., Mom's longtime childhood friend and the oldest, at 88 years, would forget her reading glasses. That left Lois, the youngest, an East Coast liberal with straight white bangs across her forehead, often wearing a black tunic sweater, to preserve the "reading group" identity. She chose *New Yorker* or *Atlantic Monthly* articles to read aloud to the others. On many Fridays, drinking sherry and catching up were the order of the day.

"Isn't Betty in town, Mom?"

My mother used to make suggestions to me, veiled as questions. As a child, if I said I didn't have enough friends, her answer was, "What about that darling Debbie?" All I had wanted was a sympathetic ear to listen to my whining. I tried to curb my impatience with Mom, my urge to shake her up by saying, "Figure it out yourself." I was getting cranky. I changed course. "You sound tired, Mom."

"I'm worn out from watching your father go downhill. Straight. Down. Hill. You know what happened yesterday?"

I pushed my chair back from the computer, took off my reading glasses, and set them on my papers so that I wouldn't be tempted to work as we talked. "What happened?"

"Yesterday your father didn't come down to breakfast. It was completely quiet upstairs. I called, 'George, George.' No answer. So I went up. He was sitting on a chair in his shorts with one sock on and his shirt lying on his lap. He was staring blankly at the window—not out the window. Perfectly still like a statue. He didn't turn to look at me. So I said, 'Are you all right, George?' He said he was thinking about what to wear. Thinking about what to wear? He's gotten dressed every day of his life without any trouble."

"Something's really wrong with Dad. He seems to be lost in his own mind."

"This man isn't my George, Susan. I don't like him calling me a 'frost' or a 'fraud.' And I hate what this does to our life."

As Mom spoke, the Alzheimer's warning signals flashed in my mind, in brilliant neon colors so garish they sickened me in the pit of my stomach. I chastised myself for not putting two and two together sooner: Dad's confusions, failure with numbers, insecurities, and "weekend cash" hidden so that only Judy could find it. Not just a single sign, but a whole family of indicators. As far as I knew, my father had never called any of us names. Now Dad's nastiness toward Mom announced a change. Mom could no longer endure her husband's failures. She was showing the telltale exasperation of caregivers' symptoms: fatigue, impatience, anger, and despair. 'So we're off on this Alzheimer's journey again,' I said to myself. 'Oh no, oh please, God, spare us, spare me,' I prayed silently.

"I think, Mom, we should have a professional evaluate Dad, you, and the whole situation. What do you think?"

"No one else can handle this. We don't need a stranger trying to figure us out." Mom's tired voice turned feisty. "Who would you get?"

"An organization that assesses and manages the needs of old people. They would assign a social worker."

"Your father would have to agree. I don't want anyone snooping around here or trying to change us. Not after all these years."

"Mom, what if I make an appointment for someone to come over? I think Missy and George will agree that it's a good idea. We'll find somebody—an experienced person—to give you ideas of how to organize your life with Dad and how to get some relief."

"I don't think we need it." Then she paused and changed her mind, as if in a nanosecond she glimpsed relief, even the possibility of good times: "I'm certainly not having any entertainment these days. Anything would be better than this."

I arranged for a professional evaluation of Dad and was with my parents for the future social worker/care manager's initial interview because

I, too, would be working with her, just as we had worked with Sharon for John's family. On her intake visit, Donna hurried into my parents' living room—her sleek black hair in a boyish cut, her features narrow and pointed, her navy suit with a tailored jacket over slim trousers, and high heels that barely made her as tall as Mom. Donna, edgy and sleek, perched on a flowered chintz armchair.

Clipboard in hand, fast questions at the tip of her tongue, Donna ran through my parents' daily habits: three meals a day with tea in the afternoon and cocktails before dinner, books rather than television, and so on. I watched her note which partner answered which question and assess how much my father stumbled, repeated himself, or deferred to my mother. Donna raced on to inquiries that would, I imagined, reveal their ability to cope with finances, healthcare, household management, hygiene, and medications. I worried that my very private parents would find her questions too intrusive, as she investigated corners of their lives that I had never before heard articulated. She jiggled her foot in its chic, pointy shoe. Her no-nonsense-I've-heard-it-all-before manner captivated my father, so he didn't flinch when she announced that she would return in a week to clean and organize his desk with him. The initial interview lasted about an hour. After the social worker left, Mom made no comment about Donna's high heels with pants suit—a combination she deplored.

Dad and Mom signed a contract that spelled out Donna's possible services—counseling for Mom, organization of the household along with more helpers as needed, and advice on future assisted living or nursing home placement for Dad. Her charge in 1999 was about $75 per hour. The 2008 fee for care managers' initial Cost of Care Planning consultation, which might have included an assessment of Medicare/Medicaid, financial strategies, and nursing home options ranged from $50 to $300.

In the middle of 1999, Dad's doctor requested several tests to eliminate possible causes of his deteriorating memory and cognitive functions. These included a blood test for his vitamin B-12 level and a CAT scan or MRI of his brain on the long chance that there might be a tumor. Because Paul had had similar tests, I understood that through such tests, doctors could eliminate several causes of a person's mental and behavioral changes. At that time, doctors at Washington University School of Medicine in St. Louis had about a 90-percent success rate in diagnosing Alzheimer's disease among living patients, through elimination of other causes and administration of tests they created. Their diagnosis could only be confirmed after a patient's death by a brain autopsy. Assessment tests—some written, some by interviews—include a range of cognitive, memory, and reasoning tasks to determine skills essential for independent daily living, such as a sense of time and place and the capacity to perform routine activities.

Mom concurred that Dad should have blood tests and a brain scan; she accompanied him, yet she didn't understand that the negative test results were not good news. Instead, the results showed no discernible reason for Dad's behavioral changes, cognitive decline, and increasingly hostile personality. The doctor concluded that 90-year-old Dad was, in all likelihood, a victim of Alzheimer's disease.

—⁂—

Over a three-day period in July, while John and I were on vacation in Michigan, Dad called me eleven times about his auto insurance. The first time he phoned, I was reading *Bridget Jones's Diary* and chuckling to myself. I answered the phone in the cottage living room:

"Chickadee, it's about my auto insurance on our two cars. I have a bill here due at the end of August. What do I do about it?"

"Well, Dad, you'll need to send it to the trust officer for payment."

"You do know that I have two cars even though I don't drive? The second one is for your brother or for an emergency if the first is out of commission. What do I do about insurance?"

"Do you have any questions about the papers from the company, Dad?" As soon as I'd said it, I realized how thoughtless I was to ask because everything financial was now one big question for him. "It's a great day here, Dad. It's your kind of north wind with a bright blue sky."

"Any freighters out on the lake?" Dad used to study the horizon through binoculars. He tracked oil tankers, Great Lakes freighters, and sailboats from the Mackinaw-Chicago yacht race.

"I'll take a look and let you know. Just save the insurance stuff till I get home. Or show it to George or Missy—they're both in town now. There's plenty of time."

"Okay. Good idea. Are you and John getting along well? How are the blueberries? We'll talk later."

His next call came a couple of hours later. I had moved to the old wicker chaise longue on the porch. I was dozing when the ring of the cordless phone jarred me.

"Hello."

"Chickadee, I have a question about my auto insurance."

"Fire away, Dad." I leaned back on the pillows.

"Now the form lists two cars: a Chevy and a Buick. That's what I have, isn't it?"

"Right."

"But the insurance cost is different for each car. What should I do?"

"Well, Dad, that's because one car is older than the other."

From his nap upstairs in the cottage, John called out: "Who are you talking to on the phone?"

"Is that someone calling you? I don't want to keep you. I just wanted to check on this auto insurance."

"Okay, Dad. Don't worry. Show it to George or Missy, or wait till I get home, or send it to your man at the bank." I forgot that all these options were too complex for an Alzheimer's patient. In my mellow Pentwater spirit, I'd heard Dad's polite voice and grammatical sentences. For a moment on that day, a day he would have loved, Dad was present in Michigan as the rational, curious, sweet person who had showed me how to focus the binoculars on boats on the far horizon and how to grip a tennis racket for a backhand shot. Then there were our family's beach parades organized by Dad, who believed any day was a great day for a parade. I'd temporarily forgotten that my role was now showing him how to read an insurance bill and choosing a course of action. I missed Dad in Michigan—his voice discussing literature with me; his stack of foreign policy books and spy novels (John le Carré was a favorite); his steady, accurate tennis game; his interest in me and who I had grown to be.

As I fielded car insurance questions from my father, I remembered how he'd engineered family celebrations in Michigan. In their elementary school years, Ellen, Will, and Carol had scampered down the steps from our cottage and pattered along the boardwalk to Mom and Dad's cottage just four cottages north. The sound of their bare feet faded as they started up the flight of stone steps to visit their grandparents.

Breathless from the climb back up the steps to our cottage, Ellen led her siblings. She announced, "Grandpa says we're going to have a parade on the beach tomorrow night." I'd thought of those parades as I listened to Dad's confusion over the phone.

"Where's the old flag?" Will had asked. "Grandpa wants us to carry one."

Carol, the youngest, chimed in: "I wish I'd brought my trombone."

"We could bang pots and pans," Ellen suggested.

"Do you think we'll be able to play ball afterward?" said Will.

"After the parade and s'mores," Ellen said. "And we don't even need shoes, Grandpa said."

My father had a fetish about bare feet. He hated to be barefoot anywhere, even on the beach. He tried to prevail on all of us to bow to his quirk. We never did.

Phone receiver to my ear, I pictured a long-ago evening toward sunset. We had gathered on the beach, instructions having traveled along the boardwalk to bring marshmallows and long forks for the beach fire after the parade. Will had found an old flag in the closet under the front stairs of our cottage. Dad rolled up the cuffs of his khakis, pulled his white tennis hat down against the low sun, and called us together. As the family leader, he prescribed that evening's marching order—oldest to youngest, youngest to oldest, or family groups together. We fell into line with good humor and an occasional twinge of embarrassment, as we marched along the water's edge. Except for Dad, we were a barefooted, ragtag group that never stayed long in formation. Dad would compose a chant as we walked:

"Here we are, all together, all our family, marching along, marching along, marching along on the beach in Pentwater. Here we are, all together...."

Mom had smiled at Dad as we paraded, chanted, and banged, tramping 100 yards north then back to our beach. Walt and John, the sons-in-law, and Paul and Silvia, if they were visiting, must have found our family celebration, accompanied by banging pots and a tuneless chant, to be odd, if not mad, but they all marched along.

My mind wandered back to the 1970s, when our children had broken parade ranks for a whiffle ball game or a beach chase; after the parade they would sprint into the lake for an evening swim. Later, in the 1980s, as adolescents, the kids shuffled through parades, rolling their eyes or muttering at the shame of a family that behaved like this on a beach where others might see them and wonder what sort of a cult they belonged to. Then, with a combination of pride and curiosity about outsiders' reactions, one after another, our children introduced boyfriends, girlfriends, and houseguests to family parades. Willingness to participate in this silly yet important ritual was a test—in fact, the ultimate test item for a suitor who came into our Pentwater world. Suitors, houseguests, and in-laws needed to pass the test of a family parade led by Dad, our tall, white-haired patriarch, chanting along the shore of Lake Michigan—simply by marching with us.

I turned toward the lake to watch the afternoon north wind kick up white-capped waves. The thud of waves on the sand resounded up the dunes onto our porch. I missed Dad, who was still alive but not the same person. His legs were now as thin as sticks, too weak and brittle for tennis or for beach parades. His head of white hair often had the look of a mad King Lear. Names slipped away before he could catch them. His once-keen intellect could no longer decipher foreign affairs or numbers. Instead, his language, clear and correct, often depicted an unknown world with few recognizable landmarks: robbers, Russian directors, buried treasure, long-ago church friends, hidden silver, and conspiracies. Dad's strange topics of conversation, laced with paranoid concerns so unlike him even a year or so ago, clearly signaled that Alzheimer's disease was kicking in.

"Okay, Dad," I said, "We'll keep in touch."

"John," I called up to my husband, "I was talking to my Dad. He's showing his age. I'm sad. Maybe I'll come and take a nap."

But the phone rang again and again, until at last Dad accepted that the car insurance could wait. July in Pentwater was fast spinning itself out.

—✍—

I found a teaching substitute for myself one day in September so that I could drive my parents to a Planned Parenthood luncheon, where Mom was to receive an award. Mom looked vibrant in a sapphire blue suit that heightened the white of her hair, which she had had styled at a special appointment the day before. Dad had the air of a rumpled English squire with his tweed sport coat and his cane.

As we crossed the parking lot, Mom walked ahead because she was steadier than Dad and anxious to begin her role as an awardee at the meeting. With one hand on his cane, Dad reached into his jacket pocket with the other.

"Do you see this piece of paper, Chickadee?"

"Yes, Dad."

Dad stopped, unfolded the paper, and said, "It's your mother's name. I asked her to write it down for me." He spelled it out, "D-O-R-O-T-H-Y. Now I won't forget it."

How on that sparkling autumn day, on that day of celebration, could this happen? I felt a chill of sadness as I put one foot in front of the other.

I took Dad's free arm and guided him to one of the head tables, where we sat with Mom and the other honorees.

The luncheon chair rang a fork against a glass. "I'd like to invite our first award winner forward. She needs no introduction because she has been a leader in this organization almost since its beginnings. How many of us has she mentored! For how many of us has she been a beacon in the fight for women's reproductive rights! Please welcome. . . ." And she called Mom's name.

Dad watched, matching Mom's public name to the slip of paper in his pocket, the name whose letters must have melted through tweed, old oxford cloth, the pores of old man's skin into his blood, flowing up through his thin trunk, his spine repaired by surgeries through his neck, to the brain that would construct the letters like a scrambled word game into the name of the woman he had been married to for more than sixty years. He stared at her as she held the award and smiled for a photographer.

The gathering of women applauded.

Mom spoke, her voice projecting to a vast meeting room of women sitting at round tables.

"Humble gratitude," she said. "Humble gratitude is my overwhelming emotion because I could never have fought these battles without all of you, each and every one." She held her head high and smiled, as if she were posing for a theater audition portrait in the 1930s.

I wondered what Dad saw and heard, whether he remembered Mom at her full force, when she first fought to change Missouri law so that teachers could remain on the job once married or when she sought a face-to-face meeting with the Roman Catholic cardinal in St. Louis in hopes of opening an abortion dialogue. Dad peered at his coffee like a seer searching for a message, for directions.

A second time, we applauded Mom, who bowed her head, then stepped back to her place and patted Dad's arm. He lifted his head in recognition of her touch and began to drink his coffee.

As we threaded our way through the crowd after the luncheon, Dad's cane clump-clumped to make a path. Several of my friends stopped me:

"What a mother!"

"You have quite a role model."

Crossing the parking lot, Mom held her plaque tight and acknowledged many compliments and congratulations. Dad held my arm with one hand, his cane with the other.

"Quite a day, Chickadee," he said, as if he couldn't recall what set this day apart. I ached for my father.

"Well, Susan, it must be quite something to be your mother's daughter!" a friend called out to me.

"It is. It is." Quite something. A quilt of memories—not appliquéd in a looped wedding ring pattern but a patchwork of scraps. Bright patches, souvenirs of a trip alone with Mom to Greenwich Village when I was about 16 years old, where she bought me a blue and green woven and fringed Panamanian sash, as radical a bit of fashion as I'd ever owned. I remembered the colored shapes of moments when I bragged to her about our children, when I told her how pleased I was to see an article I'd written published in a journal. Mom had encouraged and praised me as a mother and as an academic. Dark threads stitched, too, through the quilt: Mom's harsh words about relatives or criticisms of friends, her boredom and melancholia as she tried to engage Dad to lift her spirits, to help her gather energy yet again for her dance of civic leadership. I rejoiced for my mother that day. The applause from women honoring her for more than fifty years of service gave her the recognition she had earned.

"Give me a hand here, Chickadee," Dad said, as he backed up to the front seat of the car. "You take my cane while I swing my legs in."

Mom set herself and her award in the back seat.

"Well, how did you like the whole thing?" she asked, but before either of us could answer, she said, "It was thrilling, wasn't it?"

—⁂—

Early on September 28—I remember the date because I awoke thinking of our son, Will, whose 31st birthday it was—Dad called.

"Good morning. How are you, Dad?"

"Just fine. Doing fine. I fell out of bed."

"What, Dad? Are you okay?"

"I'm moving fine," he said. "I have a black eye and some blood. I'm going to call the eye doctor."

"Wait, Dad. Can I talk to Mom before you do anything?"

Mom came on the phone: "Actually, I've decided to wait for Judy to see what she thinks."

"Mom, tell me Dad's symptoms."

"He has blood coming out of his ear and his eye. It's really nothing. I am a little uneasy."

"When will Judy be there?"

"Any moment."

"Okay, Mom. Keep Dad quiet. It doesn't sound as if you need an eye doctor. How about the internist? Keep me posted. Call me at work."

'Prayers,' I said to myself, and 'hang on, hang in,' as I watched my father, like Paul, fall down, crash down, down as far as Alzheimer's disease could go. 'Take my hand, precious Lord.'

—∞—

Dad's ear was badly cut, his eye blackened. When he fell out of bed, he had caught his arm in the cord of his bedside lamp, one of a pair flanking the big double bed. The lamps were shaped like tall, wrought-iron bushes, their metal branches painted bright yellow with green leaves stretching out, as if to invite birds to nest or lemons to sprout. The tone was gala Mexican or maybe Tuscan—expansive for the bedroom Mom cherished. She and a decorator friend, Elizabeth, had painted the walls a vivid mustard yellow; French doors opened onto a balcony with window boxes planted each spring with red and purple petunias—a mixture of colors like a Matisse painting of Provence. For the far end of the room facing the balcony, Mom and Elizabeth selected a chaise longue and a slipper chair, both covered in pale silk. Mom loved to settle into the chaise to read or file her nails.

When Dad fell, that lamp with its sharp metal leaves pulled over, and several leaves jabbed his head. In the tangle of cord, leaves, and Dad's limbs, a piece of metal cut his ear.

Dad's late September fall led to a hospital stay, where he was delirious the entire time. When he returned home, he was still confused and hostile. His doctor recommended home health aides for at least 20 hours a day. At first, instead of hiring aides, Mom asked Judy, the housekeeper, to stay later in the evenings and expanded her duties to help look after Dad. Judy drove him on errands—he always needed new batteries for his old flashlights that never worked. She prepared lunch and dinner, cleaned up the dishes, served as primary searcher for the many things Dad misplaced, such as glasses, cash, and pieces of mail. Judy stayed with Dad while Mom went grocery shopping or to her Friday reading group. George always spent April, May, and September in Italy; Missy had a demanding public relations job with a less flexible routine than mine. My schedule as a full-time university teacher appeared flexible, in that I met my classes and kept student-advising office hours at certain times. For the rest of each day, I set my own timetable for course preparation and writing and reading duties. Thus, I was usually Mom and Dad's "go to" person. I felt overwhelmed.

By the end of September 1999, I was on overload. Although I kept my cell phone turned off at work, I often returned home to find voice messages. Every phone call from my parents put me on edge. I couldn't figure out how the various pieces of my life could possibly fit together— my parents' house, healthcare, and well-being; evenings with John, my teaching and writing work, and staying in touch with our children. John visited Silvia by himself several times a week, and we often visited her together on weekends. I was suffering managerial stress.

That September I had arthroscopic knee surgery. I was in physical therapy with a program of exercises to do at home. My close friend, Helen, was diagnosed with cancer and a few weeks later was assaulted and robbed in her own house nearby; I never felt I spent enough time with her. At the university, my friends Minette and Allen were dealing with major illnesses. I was worried, too, about our daughter, Ellen, who had moved to Connecticut for her work, because she had been prescribed bed rest in the last trimester of her first pregnancy. I didn't have enough time to do anything adequately, such as be a good friend, a focused professional, a helpful mother, or John's closest friend and wife. I resented spending twenty minutes on the knee exercises.

That year, nonetheless, I pushed myself to appreciate an Indian summer that stretched from early October through mid-November with golden days and cool nights. The weather and Judy's presence allowed Mom to drive to the grocery store two or three times a week, a diversion she enjoyed, though she often bought nothing but a tomato, some chocolate, or a small bouquet of flowers. She had always delighted in the sensuous array of colors, smells, textures, and promised tastes that a market offered. My knee recovery progressed; my classes went well, especially a seminar on teaching foreign languages I offered to incoming graduate students. As I look back on that fall, I recognize that I was steeling myself for the rough waters ahead.

Dad recovered from his fall. Thanks to home physical therapy (covered by Medicare), he was steadier and more confident on his feet than he had been in a while.

Physically he was better, but he became increasingly delusional, a symptom typical of Alzheimer's disease, and I became the scapegoat for his paranoia. I accompanied Mom and Dad on a doctor's visit:

Dad began, "Doctor, isn't the daughter supposed to be the loving one?"

The doctor said, "Could you explain what you mean, please?"

"My daughter here decided that she would let me, the son of a bitch, rot," my father answered.

"Tell me a little more, please," the doctor said.

"My daughter here has conspired to take my house away. I don't live there any more."

The doctor looked respectfully at my father. "Sometimes, sir, people with your condition don't remember well and confuse important things. I think you're doing that. You do still live in your house."

I swallowed hard to keep back my tears.

—⁂—

On a late fall afternoon, I arrived at Mom and Dad's house after teaching my graduate seminar. They were in the living room in front of a freshly lit fire, my mother in a blue upholstered chair she called the shepherd's chair, my father in a low flowered armchair, his long legs stretched to the hearth. Their Siamese cat YumYum meowed at me from a rose-colored throw on the end of the couch. The three of us formed a triangle as I sat in a second flowered armchair on the other side of the fire. I leaned my head back against the chair, spread my arms, and sighed:

"Long seminar. Big teaching concepts that are hard for the students." I closed my eyes in the warmth from the fire.

"Did you know that my silver is missing?" my father answered.

"Your silver, Dad?"

"It's all gone." Dad folded his knees in, stared at me. "Even though I buried it in Sever Park."

"I wanted to tell you about these ideas we worked on today in my seminar, about how you best learn and teach language."

"And I'm telling you, my silver is gone."

"George, please, Susan drove all the way out here after work." My mother reached for a covered glass candy dish. She lifted the top: "Why don't we have some chocolate?"

My father bit into a chunk of milk chocolate. My mother broke a piece in half. Yummy stirred on the couch.

"The debate," I was in earnest now, as if repeating my seminar opener, "is whether students learn better by listening and hearing first or by jumping in to try speaking right away. That's the debate."

Mom rearranged the chocolate in the dish with the tip of her forefinger, put the top back on. "That's interesting. I can tell it interests you."

"What interests me is your board of directors, Susan." My father's tone was icy. "All those directors you have who probably helped steal my silver."

My neck, my arms, my posture grew taut. The fire crackled, its sparks popped onto the hearth, its forest fragrance scented the room with comfort.

"Dad, do you want to know about how complicated it is to learn another language?" I should have known better—not this Dad, not even my dad of the past could comprehend my fascination with the French language. For him, foreign tongues were an embarrassment. A wanton distortion of the natural order of sounds and cadences. When questioned about one of his trips abroad, my father would answer, "It was thrilling, enlightening, except for all those people who chattered along in Turkish." Theories of language learning—not for him. He loved to study the etymological roots of English from the ancient Greek and Latin, which he'd studied in his classical education. But his ear was wooden. He couldn't sing a tune, although he grasped rhythm and could tap out a *Carmen* melody he'd learned from Mom. Dad cherished the old Presbyterian hymns, like "Rock of Ages" and "For the Beauty of the Earth," but he couldn't imitate the melodies or read the notes. As to pronouncing words from other languages, no hope, no chance, no way to convince him to purse his lips, pull his tongue into a funny position—how intimate and invasive could I get when I once demanded that he let go of his mother tongue to form a tight, puckered French "u"? I never should have expected a 90-year-old gent who was tone deaf and suffered from dementia to listen to me expound on language acquisition.

"I'm not here for languages. I want you to account for my silver that I stored in a lock box," he said. "When you say you're going to help, you don't. Nor do your directors. You're a fraud. You're a frost."

"Honestly, George, you don't need to talk to Susan that way."

"Don't get in the middle of this." Dad eyed my mother in a hard way I'd never seen before. "It's about my silver. You're a fraud too, Dorothy."

"Look, Dad, I don't know what silver, what park, or what box you're talking about."

I saw tears film my mother's eyes. She called to Yummy, "Kitty, kitty, come sit on my lap." Yummy stretched, hopped onto my mother's lap, and licked at bits of milk chocolate dotting the front of her sweater.

"Okay, Mom and Dad, I'm headed home before it gets dark. Your night nurse will be here soon. Are you set for dinner?"

"You don't have to go right away, do you, Chickadee?" The blue of my father's eyes lit up in the firelight, his jaw relaxed as he called me his pet name.

I gathered my coat and my purse. As my father bid me goodbye from the back door, he called out, "Remember, Chickadee, that our family sticks together, sticks together the way we did on the beach in Michigan. We have to stick together."

—⁂—

At this relatively "calm," crisis-free time during Dad's decline, Mom wanted to be in charge of their lives in consultation with Dad. But Dad understood almost nothing. I knew we needed to use this period to plan next steps for Dad with Donna's help. Yet Mom was testy when I tried to discuss making a plan for Dad's care. She and my siblings contended, "Everything is okay. All will be fine. Dad will soon settle back into a semblance of his old self." My assigned role in our family was to be the overreacting pessimist. I brought to my parents' deteriorating situation the hard-won knowledge from helping John care for Paul that Dad's Alzheimer's disease would overtake him. As his caregiver, my very old mother would suffer even deeper fatigue and despair. I could see all of this, but Mom, Missy, and George seemed to want to proceed slowly. They acknowledged that Dad needed some extra care, but they were not ready to accept that he had Alzheimer's or some form of dementia.

Donna recommended nighttime care after my father's hospital stay. Missy found an agency to provide the services of night aides. But nurse staffing problems plagued Missy and me. We tried to manage the agency's aides to guarantee consistency and competence. Yet, at night there was a shifting team of helpers we never met. We were both frustrated.

Events, however, intervened. In early December, my parents' bank trust officer discovered that Dad's credit cards had been used extensively, his signature forged. The banker, who handled all my parents' bills, asked me if my father had bought $150 jeans or jewelry at Grandpa Pigeon's Discount Store. My father? The man who still wore tattered oxford cloth shirts and a wristwatch with a faded cotton band—I laughed out loud!

At first, Missy, our parents, and I were unable to reconstruct which aide had used the cards. My parents' fear was palpable. After a consultation with Donna, we decided that our only alternative was to fire all the nighttime aides and the agency providing them. We agreed to prosecute when the police found the perpetrator. That left a frightened and vulnerable Mom and Dad with no nighttime help.

Finally, we were able to identify the aide by comparing the credit card use dates with the provider agency's records. We learned that an aide had given Mom and Dad their sleeping pills, tucked them into bed, and raided Dad's wallet where he kept his PIN number written on a piece of paper. She left them asleep for her shopping escapades. The aide had visited several cash machines on repeated occasions, filled her car with gas many times, and Christmas shopped with Dad's bank cards. Mom and Dad were not responsible for illegal charges on their cards, yet they felt violated by this breach of trust. The perpetrator was apprehended, convicted (this was not a first conviction), and sentenced.

Missy, George, and I now recognized that this moment was indeed pivotal. Our parents were deeply frightened by the ease with which they had been victimized, and accepted that they needed increased care. We relied on Donna's expertise as we began to consider the alternatives for Dad and for Mom. I remembered the lesson that in Alzheimer's cases, the primary caregiver suffers at least as much as the patient. With hindsight, I recognized that Silvia's emergency room visit for an arthritis attack, one of many such visits, and her fall on the eve of Paul's placement in a nursing home all indicated the toll that caregiving stress had taken on Silvia. The madness, unpredictability, and disruption unwittingly caused by Paul, and now by my father, flattened their caregivers like a fast-moving tornado. At the same time, as an Alzheimer's patient, my father would lose almost all memory, recall, and coherence. I knew this from Paul and from consulting books and pamphlets, such as *The 36-Hour Day* and *The Encyclopedia of Alzheimer's Disease.* The latter points out that many people in the disease's middle stage "become unable to remember major aspects of their lives," exhibit "delusional behavior," and become "obsessive and anxious" (183).

As Dad displayed more signs of middle-stage disease, such as disrupted sleep and irritability, placement became inevitable. For all of us, Donna was central to our well-being; her extensive experience and thoughtful words reassured me. She visited Alzheimer's facilities, prepared Mom for Dad to move to a nursing home, and coached us all.

The local Alzheimer's Association provided detailed information about facilities with Alzheimer's or memory units. In 2009 in the St. Louis area, a semiprivate room, such as Paul and my father had, might range from $4,625 to $8,000 per month or from $55,500 to $96,000 per year, depending on the level of care needed. (Back in 1999, a placement nearby, close enough so that Mom could have driven herself to visit Dad, would have cost about $70,000 per year.) The expenses for Mom's life in the house with Judy as chief aide-de-camp were a known quantity. While my mother might have benefited from Paul and Silvia's experience, she was a go-it-alone person in what she considered private family matters. Usually proud and secretive, Mom, nonetheless, allowed Donna to guide her. Thanks to their drive and intelligence, Dorothy and Donna bonded.

While none of the four parents anticipated the cost of being stricken with Alzheimer's disease over a long period, our families were fortunate to have adequate financial resources for excellent elder care. Donna presented three possibilities to my parents: 1) Continue with their housekeeper, Judy, as daytime helper and wait for a precipitating crisis. 2) Hire a new group of around-the-clock nurses' aides at home. For a crew of certified nurse assistants (CNAs), in 1999 the cost would have been $13 per hour or about $114,000 per year for full-time care. Ten years later, in 2009, the hourly CNA charge ranged from $18.50 to $19.25 per hour or about $162,000 per year for 24-hour care. We would have had to supplement the CNAs with household help because Mom was no longer strong enough to do the housekeeping. 3) "Placement" for my father, leaving

Mom alone in a large house on an isolated lane without her beloved spouse. All were imperfect solutions. There seemed to be no acceptable solution to being very old, needful, and dementia-ridden.

In contrast with that dismal November of credit card theft and placement decisions, a round, healthy Devon Joseph, Ellen's first baby and our first grandchild, was born in Connecticut two days after Thanksgiving 1999.

And then, in December, I thought I would become as crazy as my father, who was both paranoid and dependent. His cheerful but unrelenting calls made me detest the telephone. On Judy's days off, Mom grew desperate with worry about what to serve for dinner and whether to leave Dad alone while she went to the grocery store. While Dad and Mom were on a downhill slope, my siblings and I also showed signs of caregiver stress—impatience, lack of sleep, anger, and anguish. (These details relevant to caregivers are spelled out in the book, *Mayo Clinic on Alzheimer's Disease*, 167). I felt the need for protective armor to shield me from blows to my psyche, my brain, my spirit, my self.

Every morning one week, Dad called at about 8 a.m., as I was hurrying to leave for work. He started each call by saying he didn't know where he was. He was all alone. Who would take care of him? One day he planned to call the police, he said, because "Surely they could help a homeless man." I mourned his plight—the plight of a man who had outlived his time. Another day, he thought that I should take him to his sister Jane's funeral (she had died twenty years before). One day he phoned to tell me that a pregnant man was taking care of him.

In the midst of surreal conversations with Dad and consultations with Mom and my siblings, I tried to summon up the father who had nurtured me, especially through my adolescence in the 1950s. Perhaps, I surmised, I could hold steady in my new role as parent to my own father by clinging

to the memories of his wise support as I grew up. I remembered the Dad
who undertook my training for conversations on dates with boys, the Dad
who instructed me in how to weave my way through the world.

"I have trouble, Dad, talking to these boys. I don't know what to say,"
I had said when I was 15.

Dad got out a yellow legal pad: "Chickadee, let's make a list of
topics."

We brainstormed. Dates were on Friday and Saturday evenings with
invitations expected by Wednesday. By Thursday, my Dad and I began
my weekend preparation.

He jotted down good topics: 1) New movies: "The Robe" was popular;
"Blue Moon" was censored. 2) Sports: I could handle football because
I liked watching George, who was a high school star. I played varsity
basketball, also a good topic. 3) Summer plans or past vacations: Here I
had to be careful. One summer I broke up with my local boyfriend, our
high school's football captain and class president, in favor of an out-of-
town camp romance. When classes resumed that fall, the boys at school
shunned me for awhile. 4) Let the boys talk about themselves.

"Over all," Dad advised me, "number four is the best topic."

At one session, Dad showed me a card in his shirt pocket; he had
noted his own topics for discussion at his lawyers' lunch meeting. Sometimes he wrote "joke" with a word or two to remind him of the punch
line.

"I'll report on Sunday morning," I promised my father. Occasionally,
my date and I slow-danced, arms draped over each other's shoulders. No
talk was necessary. I fudged those reports.

—∿—

Early one morning during that week of bizarre calls, Dad began,
"When will you take me home?"

"Dad, you *are* at home."

He went on, "Well, Chickadee, you keep saying I'm at home. But when will you take me home?"

"You are living in your own house, Dad, on Ballas Road."

He continued, "I'm old, and you need to help me by letting me go home. Can't you organize it so I can go home?"

"Uh, huh," I said.

"About one hundred people in the USA tell me I'm at home," my dad said. "But everyone else knows that I'm not. Why don't you understand? You're not very humane or kind."

"Where do you mean by home?"

"With my mother in heaven."

"You mean your mother who is dead and in heaven?"

"Yes, I want to go home to my mother and father and sister in heaven, with all the nice people from Westminster Church, like the Hanfords. Don't you want to go home to your parents?"

"I understand you, Dad." I wished with all my heart that I could help him go home to be with the old friends and family who had died before him. He was pleading with me to lend a hand to an old man with an unsteady gait, as he stepped on the slippery rocks to cross the stream to the other side. I imagined he longed to recuperate what he thought he had lost: his beloved wife, the young and lovely Dorothy dear; his house, which had taken on castle-like proportions in his fragmented memory; the corporate board of directors, once the nexus of his professional world; the silver-plated Campbell family teapot from Ireland. This was the stuff of an old man's life: scattered, confused, conflated, hard won, ever precious, begging to be rediscovered on the other side—if only his Chickadee would help him over the slippery stepping stones.

How could I reconcile this miserable old man, who begged for help to go home to heaven, with my father, who had never wanted to be beholden to anyone?

On Friday morning that week, Dad telephoned.

"Could you come pick me up?"

"Where are you, Dad?"

"In Effingham, Illinois," he answered.

"Effingham?"

"Yes. I'm in Effingham," he said.

For a moment, I thought my father might have gotten himself to Effingham, Illinois, somehow. Everyone in our family yearns for Effingham because it's the turning point, the place where we turn true north toward Pentwater. We head away from the flat fields of Illinois, where the occasional pumping oil derrick breaks the green lines of soy crops and knee-high corn. North past Kankakee, Pesotum, Neoga, hurtling on around Chicago, veiled to our left in industrial haze. The Chicago exits remind us that the vast blue lake—our inland ocean—is right over there, if we could pierce through the concrete towers, warehouses, and commercial streets full of fast-food restaurants. Beyond the urban landscape lies Lake Michigan.

As our family headed north to Pentwater, we never ate lunch at a fast-food place. No, no, my father had prescribed a picnic for as long as I could remember. I recalled our 1952 drive to Michigan, when I was a wretched giant of a 13-year-old, at my full height, bone thin, with unruly blonde hair. At that and other picnics during my early teens, I was a pain. I considered myself too fat to accept potato chips, disdained the hard-boiled eggs Dorth had prepared the day before (which George cracked against his forehead), and refused to eat even a corner of a brownie.

Past the nexus of intersecting highways at Effingham, legs stretched, car refueled, the remains of lunch stowed in the picnic basket, we rolled toward Pentwater, with Effingham behind us.

Overhearing my Effingham conversation and sensing my wonderment about my father's whereabouts, John suggested that I hang up and call my parents' house.

Mom answered the phone. I asked, "How's Dad today?"

"Oh," she said, "I'm down here making coffee. Your father's upstairs getting dressed."

—⁓—

Missy held a midday Christmas dinner for our family, at first around her Christmas tree in the living room, then at a long table set with white linens and shiny silver for the celebration. I sat on my father's right. In honor of the holiday, he wore a fine, gray herringbone suit, one of his ancient oxford cloth shirts, and a striped tie. The slight slope of his shoulders emphasized his thin frame. His hands held steady on the back of his chair as my sister invited us to say grace, Dad's grace, the blessing he had taught us as children, his lifelong words of thanksgiving, of connecting the moment of our shared table with the Lord's bountiful nature. Though he never expressed his beliefs explicitly, Dad acknowledged God's grace in our family's parades on the Michigan beach, in the flowering of spring lilacs at his brick gate, in the leafing out of the stately sweet gum trees on his lawn—all were bits of grace from a higher being. Dad stood sloped, unwavering, head bowed as my sister began:

"Lord, make us thankful for all our blessings . . . "

Our voices prayed together—nieces, siblings, partners, and Mom, whose every syllable rang clearly.

". . . and keep us ever mindful of all thy teachings and of the needs of others. Amen."

Dad reached for my chair to pull it out. Dishes circulated—the turkey carved into slices, bright green parsley at the corners of the platter; dressing fragrant with onions and sage; our family's traditional corn pudding; and cranberry sauce, which I love more than anything else in the meal.

I picked up my fork. My father looked at his full plate, and he paused, out of sync with rest of us. His gaze stopped on his food, seemed to lose focus. Softly, without turning his head, he said,

"Chickadee, will you please cut my food for me?"

Around me, the party chattered, chewed, asked for seconds. But for me, the party stood still. My sense of celebration, my anticipation of the tart cranberry sauce, my curiosity about Missy's plans for her house in Colorado, my own tales of our newly wed children and first grandchild— all froze with my father's gentle request. Please help me: I can't do it I'm not able I'm not as I appear, for my hands cannot grip cannot function cannot cannot cannot, I cannot really take care of myself any more at all. And I want to go home.

I reached over to his plate and cut his turkey—white meat and dark— into bite-sized pieces. I laid his fork at the ready.

No one else noticed. This was my dad's last Christmas.

8

Perils
2000

On a gray January day, the Seven Gables Inn restaurant enfolded Mom and me in scents of garlic along with cigarette smoke from the bar. We leaned in to talk to each other, surrounded by people doing business over lunch. I'd phoned Mom to ask her to meet me for lunch, and she'd suggested this restaurant, a favorite of hers and Dad's. Judy was at home with Dad.

"Donna called me yesterday," I told my mother.

"She called you?" Her tone was one of suspicion.

"Yes. She asked me to talk to you face to face. A bed for a male resident is available in the nursing home that you and she liked best."

Mom dropped her head into her hands. She was wearing an olive green tweed suit with a large silver brooch, an abstract sun whose rays circled a solid shining center. I stared at the pin's center as she sat, head bowed for almost the length of time allotted for silent prayers in church.

"I've lost your father, Susan. My husband has gone. Today he imagined himself in elementary school all morning."

I reached out to touch her arm. "Mom, we have to move fast—decide, reserve, and make a deposit."

"Do you know what I did yesterday? I used all my wiles to stop your father from phoning the bank to find out his balance. I coaxed him, distracted him, had Judy bake brownies."

Holding her hand, I said, "We have to decide today. Missy, George, Donna, and I think we should reserve the bed for Dad. It's a double room. This is what is available now."

I sounded calm, calmer than the beat of my heart and the empty pit of my stomach, roaring at me to forget about lunch. I had reviewed the signals of trouble for Dad and Mom—a storm building, rumbling, with occasional flashes of lightning to illuminate the double set of problems faced by the diseased person and his caregiver.

Like Paul had been, my dad was nearly incontinent; incapable of managing his own medications, a responsibility Mom had taken on with Donna's guidance; unable to read or understand numbers; suspicious and accusatory; anxious about finances and his house; and unreasonably demanding of Mom. Unlike Paul, he did not wander, nor was he physically violent. Yet, the storm clouds of more severe Alzheimer's disease were gathering on the horizon.

Like Silvia, Mom had lost patience with her husband, and her energy was low. One day a few weeks before, weary and tearful, she had phoned me. Dad was out for lunch with the Peripatetics. I recognized in her voice the indicators that "caregivers are at high risk of depression, physical illness and fatigue" (Petersen, 167). Donna also saw the impending troubles and counseled us to move quickly before Dad worsened or Mom collapsed.

"What will happen to me?" my mother asked. "I never get any sleep. I'm so tired. And the house?"

I cut my grilled sandwich into bites. "Mom, we have this offer now. Dad won't get better. Taking care of him, even with Judy, is hard on you. Too hard on you. He needs to be in a safe place with professional care."

"I didn't mean for it to be like this." She shook as she poked at her food.

"No one meant it. Dad's almost 91 years old."

"What else can we do?"

"This is the best plan, Mom."

"Then, will you talk to Donna, or will I? Who will tell your father? What will happen to me in the house?"

"So you agree? Because if you do, we'll have a lot of paperwork and some banking to arrange the initial deposit and automatic monthly payments."

"I agree." She pushed her half-eaten lunch away. "May I have some coffee? Do you have time, Susan?"

"I have time." All the time it takes, Mom, I thought, for us to decide together, even with guilt choking me, keeping me from eating, all the time you need to close the door on your long years with Dad, to salute the death that hovers over him, Mom, salute its wrenching grip on his words and numbers, on his entire being. "I need some coffee, too. I'm cold." I wrapped my arms around my chest, wondering how to ward off the cold and the sadness.

—⁓—

In mid-January, we moved Dad to the locked Alzheimer's unit of a nursing home. Donna coached Mom about telling Dad that, in fact, he would no longer live in his own house. Aware of Mom's need to rest, Donna proposed a temporary stay in the same nursing home's unit dedicated to short-term respite for caregivers. Mom would get a two-week rest, and she could walk down a few hallways to visit Dad as many times a day as she wanted. Because his unit was locked, he could not visit her.

George and I carried out the move on a brilliant January day, the north wind brisk enough to whip up white-capped waves on Lake Michigan. I drove Dad, who was cheerful, while George drove Mom. The day before, Donna had arranged Dad's side of his room with a few familiar trappings, such as a beloved multicolored afghan. His memory box, labeled "George," hung beside the door of his room and contained pictures of himself in college and in the Marine Corps, on travels with Mom, and at business functions—all to remind him of himself.

Donna helped settle Mom into her room for a two-week rest, while Dad, a nurse, and I passed through the doors into the Alzheimer's unit at the other end of the building. A cat on the couch in the common room stretched as we walked by. Dad appeared interested in these new surroundings, cooperative in giving what he could remember of his medical history, and even ready to participate in the men's club that afternoon. I swallowed hard as I filled in the blanks in his medical past. And I bit my bottom lip to keep from crying as I said good-bye. A nurse let me out of the unit.

George, Donna, and I reconvened in the lobby, where a red-striped cart with a carnival look would make popcorn later in the day during the residents' entertainment hour. I imagined a jaunty vendor hawking popcorn as if he were at the state fair. There would be the wheelchair-bound residents, the murmuring-pacing Alzheimer's victims released from their locked unit, and the dowager-humped ladies with helmets of white hair coiffed, ready for that day's gathering in the lobby.

"Your mother changed her mind. A complete about-face," Donna said.

"About what?" George asked.

"About her healthcare directive code and your dad's."

"How could she? It's all written down—no heroic medical efforts to save their lives," I said. "Dad never would agree, even now."

"She changed her code and your dad's when she signed the paperwork to admit him."

"She can't. She doesn't have the right," George said. "It was all decided by the two of them and drafted by their lawyer in their advance medical directives."

I had been so moved by Dad's vacant, cheerful acceptance of a men's club meeting in the Alzheimer's unit and by the tawdry festivity of the popcorn cart that I couldn't face a negotiation with our mother about their healthcare directive, the code that would now prescribe full efforts to save and preserve their lives if either had a health crisis. I didn't believe Mom wanted either of them to have shocks to the heart, IVs pumping life preserving fluids into senseless bodies, or artificial breathing machines. Dad was quickly disappearing into a foreign mental and emotional realm, while she, like an abandoned wraith, would haunt the spaces of their beloved house. Surely she didn't want all possible efforts to be made to extend their lives?

But she had indeed changed their directives. Printed in bold, black marker on Mom's file and on Dad's: "Full Code—Full Code."

A few weeks after his placement, Dad fell near the sofa in the unit's living room, a spontaneous fall, so the nurses said. He broke his hip. Gathered in the emergency room waiting area, George, Missy, our mother, and I were given about fifteen minutes to decide whether Dad should have hip surgery.

"You know," the doctor said, "he will never walk again if we don't operate."

I should have asked that doctor to sit down long enough for me to explain something—not about hips or walking or Medicare beds or recovery, but about the reality of life for a man nearly 91 years old with mid-stage Alzheimer's disease, who had already walked in places like Kashmir and Nepal and along the medieval pilgrimage route to Santiago de Compostela in Spain; who'd climbed peaks, slipped once in the Alps where a German mountaineer to whom he was belayed caught him and saved his life; who'd already walked through a successful career and community service with honors; who'd walked his Springer spaniel for miles, tap-tapping his cane as he went; who'd marched along the beach in Michigan well into his eighties; who'd walked the stairs in his house and the path to the mailbox, in a smaller and smaller orbit until he began to stumble and fall in the most familiar places, such as the basement stairs. I should have beseeched that doctor to tell us how it was that his magical surgery would enable my father to walk again as he had walked through his life.

The four of us listened to the doctor. Mom replied, "Please operate. We will be in the waiting room."

"When he goes to the recovery room, I'll come talk to you," the doctor said.

About what, I wondered? The pain medications Dad would need, the Medicare bed he would return to instead of the Alzheimer's unit, oh yes, and the catheter, and his program of Medicare-financed intensive physical therapy. I managed to ask before he left us, "Do you realize, sir, that the anesthesia and the shock of the surgery often worsen Alzheimer's symptoms and trigger extreme confusion?"

"We expect that," the doctor said, "but your father will be well cared for; we'll get him back on his feet."

Doctor, you don't understand, I wanted to say. His feet are narrow and light-boned for someone so tall. They can't hold him up any longer. You don't know, doctor, but my father hates to walk barefooted, even on a beach. Please allow him socks in the recovery room; he likes white wool tennis socks. And then, doctor, please notice the pressure sore on his ankle. It won't heal—not ever—because he has poor circulation below his knees. Please consider letting him rest now. But I said all of this to myself, grieving for the person who had left us a long time ago.

Dad celebrated his 91st birthday a few days after the hip surgery. George, Missy, and I visited him one after another that day. During my birthday visit, Dad said, "You know, this is my 51st birthday. I'm just like my grandfather George, who lived to age 22."

"Dad, would you like some more chocolate?" Like a child, he had smudged chocolate on his fingers and at the corners of his mouth.

"I'd love some more. It's good for an old gent."

Four days after his birthday, in the middle of the night, Dad had a massive heart attack. The nursing home went into Full Code gear, as did the ambulance attendants. When I got the call at 2 a.m., I drove fast on a starry February night, singing hymns as loudly as I could. "My faith looks up to thee, thou Lamb of Calvary, . . . be thou my guide. . . ." I was the first of the family to arrive in the emergency room, where a cardiologist met me. Then George came. And Missy. Mom arrived just as the cardiologist said, "He's having a series of heart attacks."

"Is he conscious? Will he know us?" I asked.

"Go talk to him," the doctor said.

Everything was icy white and stainless steel.

"Dad, do you hear me?"

"Chickadee. Can you help me go home?"

"I'll be right here with you, Dad."

"Can't you help me hurry home to my mother and my father?"

"We're right here with you. Go home when you're ready, Dad."

Mom had completed her respite stay and once again lived with Yummy in the family house. Judy helped her during the day. Driving to the hospital, Mom got lost, eventually located the hospital, and found us in the ER.

With his back to our mother, the cardiologist said to us: "I see your father has Full Code."

"Our mother changed it to that just recently."

"I don't think there's much we can do for your father. I'd like to wait to see what happens."

The three of us—Missy, George, and I—understood that the doctor was overriding Mom and her Full Code directive. We nodded our consensus, and he explained to Mom that Dad was having a series of heart attacks.

Those attacks wore Dad down until he became silent and calm. Death rattled through his throat and chest later that afternoon.

We held Dad's funeral on February 26 (John's birthday), in Westminster Presbyterian Church, Dad's family's church, where John and I were married. Throughout his life, Dad continued to attend Sunday services by himself once or twice a month; he served as an elder and a staunch supporter until he could no longer drive. After our parents had raised us as Presbyterians, Mom joined the Episcopal Church, where she served as a lay reader. In her Episcopalian faith, Mom found an historic ritual with elegant prayers, which she preferred to the austere Presbyterian liturgy. As for my sister and brother and me, Missy was active in a Congregational Church before her move to Colorado, George rarely attended services, and I remained a practicing Presbyterian. I'd joined a church in our neighborhood, one I could walk to on Sunday mornings.

Dad would have enjoyed his funeral. He didn't mind being at the center of a gathering, whether seated on the deck in Pentwater or at his full 6'3" in the middle of a party. A fine extemporaneous speaker, Dad was easily persuaded to make toasts. He liked to celebrate himself at his own birthday parties, occasions for speech making followed by the politician's overhead victory clasp. At a dinner party given by Mom for family and close friends in honor of his 60th birthday, Dad's toast had resembled a sermon:

"Now people ask me about my secret to long life." (Sixty had seemed old then.) "I have to answer that the best model, the best guide I know for living life is Jesus. He's the guiding principle that has worked for me. So that's my answer."

This made for some awkward silence and a pause among his secular friends. Were they to raise their glasses and say, "Here's to Jesus?" I was 30 years old at that party and surely rolled my eyes or nudged John under the table in embarrassment.

At 65, he lightened up. Newly retired from corporate life and public banquets, he began taking a sketching course at the art museum and planting tulip gardens for Missy and me. His birthday party—our family loves major birthday happenings—was formal and elegant, yet intimate, with maybe twenty-five friends and family. Again, Dad gave himself a toast:

"Now that I'm 65 and retired, I'm going to make two vows to last me to the end of my days."

Catching the twinkle in his eyes, his friends chorused, "Hear! Hear!"

"First, I'm never going to another public banquet at the Khorassan Room or any other hotel banquet facility. Never."

Everyone applauded.

"Second, I'm going to drink as much bourbon whiskey as I want."

Glasses clinked, and Dad embarked on his new campaign. Though excess was Dad's professed desire, he had only one or two drinks nightly, with such a ritual of rules that he couldn't have consumed much bourbon between ages 65 and 91. No cocktails before 6 p.m. CST, although he occasionally allowed himself and Mom to imagine being on Eastern Time with old college friends, granting 5 p.m. drinks. There were always little crackers and blue cheese or cheddar. Mom provided canned ripe olives for special occasions. Together, Dad and Mom drank their evening bourbon drinks or gin and tonics in the summer. Their second drinks were slightly lighter, with more water and a little less whiskey. That was it for alcohol consumption. Dinner came an hour later with no wine, for wine drinking seemed an affectation to them, although they enjoyed a glass at others' homes.

In their most senior years, Mom and Dad read aloud if they were alone for drinks, one on each side of the fireplace in the living room, passing tomes of Conrad, Snow, and Galsworthy back and forth, as they revisited tales from their younger days.

Dad was used to public speaking well beyond toasts. He was singled out—elected or chosen—enough times to perfect his politician's two-hands-clasped victory salute, the one he used in the Flynn Park parade. He was president of the St. Louis Bar Association, elected to a school board, ordained as a church elder, and mentioned as a possible candidate for the U.S. Congress. That clasp—like an athlete's arm pump—was part of his legacy, as the minister reminded us in his eulogy at Dad's funeral:

"George loved canoeing on Missouri rivers. And he particularly loved shooting the rapids. Some time in his youth, he'd learned to shoot them standing up in the stern of a canoe, using his paddle as a rudder or a pole.

"So George, with Dorothy seated in the bow, set out down a lively set of rapids on an Ozark stream. His canoe was the first of the group to go.

Tall George stood up on the gunwales in the stern. The canoe slapped its way through those rapids, George shifting his weight as the canoe sped through the 'V' of the water.

"As the canoe floated into the calm pool at the bottom of the rapids, George turned around—remember that he was standing—to salute his friends in their canoes. He stretched full height, gave the victory clasp over his head. And promptly lost his balance and toppled into the river." The minister smiled and looked directly at Mom and at the three of us; we could not help but smile back, as the memory of Dad falling from his full height into an Ozark stream lightened the moment.

Victories could be that way. As you pump the air with pride, you tumble into deep waters. Dad's last victory clasp, Missy reminded me after the funeral, was on his 91st birthday from his wheelchair in the large dining room of the nursing home. Four days after the balloons, the cake, and the birthday song, Dad toppled from life into death.

Though Dad had served in the U.S. Marine Corps, he had chosen the U.S. Navy hymn to close the service. We sang, "Eternal Father, strong to save, . . . O hear us when we cry to Thee, for those in peril on the sea." On the sea or an Ozark stream or Lake Michigan—when frothy waves pitch and buffet us daily and imperil our lives, we cry out. I cried out that day of Dad's funeral, along with prayers and hymns dedicated to his life, for God's help with the mothers.

On that gray rainy day, at the family plot in Bellefontaine Cemetery, Mom, surrounded by her children, grandchildren, first great-grandchild Devon, and cousins, laid a white rose on Dad's coffin.

I returned to work one week after Dad's funeral. I planned to teach the death of Flaubert's Emma Bovary in my undergraduate course called Voyages and Discoveries. In this course we read and discussed French masterworks in English to fulfill what Washington University used to call a "distribution requirement," that is, a broadening-horizons requirement for students with majors outside the humanities. There are no parallels between Emma's death and my father's, although both were preceded by hints of an imminent end. Black crows wheel in the sky over Emma Bovary's head. A bailiff arrives to make an inventory of the Bovary household goods to repay Emma's wanton expenditures, which she explains away by what Flaubert calls "a tissue of lies." No silver teapot would be spared. It takes only a minute for Emma to gorge herself with the powdery white arsenic she had purloined from the village pharmacist while he and his family ate supper in the front of their house.

I have read those ten long pages of Emma's agony over and over, beginning in my freshman year at college and on into my career, when I relived Emma Bovary's death throes every February. That passage was so accurate that only the son of a doctor, like Flaubert, who was raised in a public hospital, could have depicted the minutiae of arsenic poisoning: the sediment-filled vomit giving way to sweats, leading to a false peace just long enough for the village priest's visit. Emma's death belonged to my teaching life. During Dad's decline, my French literature and language self tried to stay focused on the job, yet thoughts of my failing father often raced across my mind.

In the February after Dad's death, my class and I plowed through the long bedroom death scene in a provincial Normandy village. The students and I lingered over Emma's startlingly sensual kiss of the priest's crucifix proffered during extreme unction. The briefer mourning scene in the family parlor stopped me. Flaubert juxtaposes the lengthy death melodrama of Emma the adulteress with a spare, ironic portrait of her husband Charles's grief. I felt like Charles, head bent to his wife's bier, without words, yet yearning for something to remember of my father, like the lock of Emma's hair that Charles covets. Suddenly, Charles's sorrow mirrored mine, and my sadness swallowed my ability to lecture that day.

"Now," I said to my students, "Please form groups of three or four. Compare and contrast the scene of Emma's death with Charles's visit to her body. I'll want some key passages on the board."

Books open, students began to reread the text. I knew to expect a loud "gross" or "yuck" when they came to the line where Flaubert describes the black liquid pouring from Emma's mouth. In contrast, my father's death was crisp and measurable. A clear buzz on the heart monitor machine announced his dying; a "Code Blue" cry in the corridor warned of full cardiac arrest.

"Maybe the family would like to take a few minutes by the body," a nurse had said. "I can crank up the bed," she offered. "Just push the call button when you are ready to leave."

A quick farewell, adieu, before the body fluids pour out their rank smells. And how long will it be until, like Charles Bovary, Mom sits in the garden after supper, holding a memento of Dad as she welcomes her own death in the twilight of a summer day?

After class, several students shyly said, "We heard from the substitute about your father. We're sorry, so sorry."

—∞—

In mid-June, Sandra, who had replaced Pat as Silvia's 40-hours-a-week caregiver, left John and me a voicemail message:

"Silvia locked herself in her bedroom. She said her purse and her checkbook were missing. So she needed to lock herself in."

Sandra, an African-American woman in her mid-fifties, had come to work for Silvia in January when Pat moved away. With thick bangs cut across her forehead and straight, shoulder-length hair, Sandra looked almost Egyptian. She spoke simply about Silvia: "She throws her pills in the trash." Then she looked down at her long shiny nails and pushed at a cuticle: "I have devised a system for the medications she takes at night after I leave."

John returned Sandra's call: "What are we going to do? Where's my mother's purse? What's wrong with her?"

"I can't tell you what's wrong, John. I just report. She burned her toast yesterday. Burned it into ashes," Sandra answered. "She's always tired. Too tired to go to exercise class."

"What can I do? What can anyone do?" John asked. "Where is her purse?"

John told me that Sandra laughed. "Her purse—this is the third time this week she's hidden it. This time it was buried up with the shawls in her closet."

"I'm at a loss, Sandra. I'm still worn out from my father," John said.

"Well, I'm 'flustrated,' too."

"What, Sandra?"

"Plain flustrated. Not having her purse makes your mother frantic, and when she acts like that, I get frantic to find the purse, and then after I finally find it, I'm just plain flustrated."

So "flustrated" became the indicator of how flustered and frustrated Sandra could get with Silvia's situation. John, too, grew flustrated as he remembered the watchwords of middle-stage Alzheimer's disease: obsessive, anxious, confused, delusional behavior (Turkington and Galvin, 183).

"I better call the Memory and Aging people at Washington U. Here we go again." John sounded tired and resigned. "Thanks for reporting, Sandra. I need your eyes and ears."

—◆—

When I was 5 years old, I had a red patent-leather purse I adored. I was as attached to my red purse as Silvia was to her tan nylon travel bags.

Mom, George, and I spent the summer on Cape Cod in a carriage house near my Aunt Mamie's place on Buzzard's Bay while Dad was deployed to the Pacific theater. Missy hadn't been born yet. I kept a few coins in my little red purse, which hung demurely on my wrist when we went to Falmouth on errands; the purse made me feel important, as if I were a grown-up. Though gasoline was rationed because of World War II, Mom and Aunt Mamie drove us to a fair on the village square.

At the fair women and children milled about; many men were away at war. Mom and Aunt Mamie chatted together, being silly and funny. Protected between them and George, with my purse on my wrist, I saw myself as one of the women of the family, mingling in with the crowd.

We stopped next to a knot of people around an organ grinder. Or, I stopped to watch. The organ grinder was exotic, frightening, with his heavy black eyebrows, sweeping mustache, and billowy white shirt. The organ hung around his neck, and he played bouncy tunes as he cranked its handle. I was more intrigued by his dancing monkey, stepping in time to the music on his two hind legs. He wore a miniature vest with gold embroidery and a jaunty cap anchored under his chin. As the monkey danced, he approached the audience and shook a tin cup, already tinkling with coins.

I stood, entranced, in the first line of spectators. I decided to offer one of my nickels, just as the bigger children and women were doing. I slid my red patent purse from my wrist and snapped open its gold clasp. When I moved my hand, the monkey darted forward. He snatched my purse, coins and all. The music swelled, and the monkey fled between people's legs into another section of the crowd. The organ grinder twirled away from me.

Tears flooded my eyes as I stared at my empty hands. I turned around to look for Mom. She wasn't behind me, nor was my aunt. I was lost in a sea of unknown women and children who hadn't seen the monkey steal my purse. The gala music cranked on across the way. And my sobbing, "Mommy, Mommy, where are you?" evaporated in the festive fair noises.

Without my red patent purse, I was alone. Frightened. The music played on. Without my purse, I was lost, just a little girl separated from her family. This foreign world swallowed me—without my purse, I felt unprotected and vulnerable. During those few moments before my mother, brother, and aunt found me, I was terrified.

—⁓—

An equally terrifying world engulfed Silvia when she "lost" her purse and its contents. Without her purse, an adult American woman's provable amalgam of herself is gone. In her battered beige bag Silvia kept an identification card, including the cold facts about when and where she was born and how tall she once stood, with a photo reflecting her direct, lively gaze. And the magic plastic cards gave her access to goods and cash of her own. Confused as Silvia was, she'd forgotten that once she had hidden her purse, its loss would torment her.

A few weeks later, Silvia limped into our house for Sunday lunch.

"What happened, Silvia?" I asked. "Come, sit down." I pulled out a chair in the dining room, where I had set the lunch table with the French doors open to the porch. The leaves of a whitebud tree moved in the June breeze.

Silvia dropped her cane beside the chair. "Nothing. I am not limping." She pulled in her chair, unfolded her napkin. "It doesn't hurt much. I crawled to a chair and pulled myself up."

"Mamma, did you fall?" John was brusque.

"It's nothing. If I feel like it, I can go downstairs to the dining room to eat. But nobody talks to me. They don't want to talk to me. It's my accent.

Nobody can understand me."

"But, Silvia." I stopped, for I knew better than trying to jolly her out of her perception. "But Silvia, what about your fall?"

John pushed his chair back and took a sip of water.

"Besides, I don't want to listen to other people in the dining room. Nothing's wrong with me. I've decided to choose my own company. I wish I had someone to talk to. My father just wanted to be by himself. It's all my fault because I don't know how to make friends," she said.

She sounded wretched as she zigzagged across her past and her self-doubts.

"Marge asked about you," I offered as a lame solace. Marge was an old friend of Silvia's who had recently moved into the same senior residence.

"Oh Marge, yes. I've never been any good at making friends. I can't remember anyone's name, so I don't know who I'm talking to. I blame myself."

And I blamed myself and John for not knowing how to lighten this lonely old lady's burdens. Nor did I have any idea how to lighten John's load. He looked all gray that summer day—hair and skin and stubbly face—in what should have been a time for him to reap the fruits of years of hard work.

"With Paul, he always did the socializing, so I saw lots of people. I feel terrible, and nobody can help. What can the doctors do? I don't see what anyone can do."

The three of us were quiet as we ate tomato salad, Fontina cheese, and crusty fresh bread; sunshine from the open doors spread over us and the remains of our lunch. For a suspended instant, I watched olive oil glistening on the salad platter, immobilized by summer inertia, Silvia's desperation, and John's flat grayness. I felt drowsy, unready for the opening salvo of dementia to begin its destruction of Silvia's brain, ready to wreck her once enthusiastic personality, her former clarity of thought.

Silvia's voice wavered through the silence: "I went to the Memory and Aging Clinic and did terribly on the test. Lots of things I'm supposed to remember and can't. I feel awful. But my leg doesn't hurt."

"Maybe the doctors can give you something to help with your mood?" I asked.

"I don't see what anyone can do to help my falls or my mood."

When John returned from driving Silvia to her apartment, his "flustration" had flattened him. He napped the rest of the afternoon. And I felt like the psalmist, "helpless and weak" when he cries out, "Save me" (Psalm 86).

—⁓—

Later in June, my mother burned the "love letters" Dad had saved from his college years before he knew Mom. She and Dad met when he returned to St. Louis to practice law. Donna had suggested that Mom burn any of Dad's files she didn't need as a step in the grieving process and, more practically, as a way to start cleaning out the attic. I had no idea whether these were love letters from a girlfriend, why Dad had saved them, nor whether Mom had "discovered" them after his death.

Dad's brief pursuit of a ballerina when he was an undergraduate in college was familiar family lore. Dad and a friend went to New York City to the ballet. They were smitten—as Dad said—by several of the dancers. They had written formal notes inviting the women to a rendezvous and had received answers. Dad never revealed anything more, which perhaps had bothered Mom. I imagined she suspected he had been alluring and witty, a kind of F. Scott Fitzgerald figure. Those letters along with other useless papers were incinerated in the stone barbecue pit at my parents' house on that June afternoon.

One day after Dad's death, as we browsed through old photos, Mom said, "I wish I'd known your father as a boy, as a lad. He was so handsome. I wish I'd known him all of his life." In those young photos of Dad, I thought his legs looked disproportionately long and his jaw, too. I didn't say anything to Mom. Yet, I found it odd that she wanted to appropriate the whole of my father into her being, which would have removed the independence and mystery and intrigue of his first 25 years.

With assertive vigor in the months after Dad died, Mom elected to have cataract surgery on one eye. After her eye had healed, Mom invited Patricia, a good friend and member of the Friday reading group, to spend the night as a houseguest. She and Mom—both opera lovers—went to a performance. Patricia had never married; she loved both my parents' company. She and Mom could reminisce about Dad—tennis, trips to Pentwater, and opera shared for decades. Mom initiated and organized this two-day event with the same verve she had planned trips and parties in years past.

Later that summer, Mom, Missy, George, and I met with our parents' attorney to consider further estate planning. Mom missed Dad at this meeting, saying, "This is serious because it involves all of Dad's worldly goods, which he had worked so hard for." She checked with the lawyer repeatedly for assurances that proposed changes in her will were what Dad would want.

The financial concepts of estate planning were difficult. Mom confirmed with her attorney that her end-of-life requests and documents were in order. She involved us three children in her thinking, although Dad had had the pertinent papers prepared. While the mood at the meeting was tense, we worked together to weigh unfamiliar family financial issues. I understood Mom's grief at the finality of the moment. Each step she took on her own—deciding to have cataract surgery, burning Dad's letters, revising the will Dad had created for her—moved her away from their intertwined lives.

—⁂—

In August 2000 while John's sister Luciana was visiting, she and John met with doctors at the Memory and Aging Project at the Washington University School of Medicine to discuss Silvia's prognosis. John suspected the outcome and was resigned. He and Luciana listened as the doctors diagnosed Silvia with Alzheimer's disease. However, Luciana questioned Silvia's diagnosis at the meeting. Her mother, she said, had never done well on tests, was nervous about them. When staff members explained the results of Silvia's various tests, Luciana accepted the findings.

Alzheimer's Association sessions and printed information warn that when out-of-town family members visit aging parents, they usually do not perceive their parents' symptoms, may deny the symptoms and diagnosis, and sometimes even try to alter arrangements, such as caregiver schedules. Moreover, John and I had repeatedly witnessed the capacity of an Alzheimer's patient like Paul to rise to a social occasion. Some patients remain largely silent, yet jovial, as they limit conversations to mannerly, long-familiar formulas. They are able to maintain their polite public demeanor well into the middle stage of the disease. Other patients listen attentively as their children, back home for a visit, fill the silence with entertaining tales of their own activities. Alzheimer's patients' remarkable "covering" or "masking" skills fuel denial by out-of-towners and by well-meaning, yet disbelieving, friends. Yet other patients invent and embroider, relating fantastical occurrences to out-of-towners who may be taken in. Even my father's "trip to Effingham" nearly convinced me that he was traveling to Pentwater.

Silvia's doctors prescribed an antidepressant. She became more cheerful and more active, attending symphony concerts, the theater, and a discussion group with clear pleasure. She didn't dwell on the bleak questions that had haunted her in spring and summer, such as, "What use am I?" She once again read political articles in the *New York Times*. At Sunday lunch, she reacted with outrage to the plight of underfed children throughout the world. As in the past, she wondered what she could do to help. Nevertheless, Silvia still became confused about dates and names; she relied on Sandra to organize her activities.

Early in the fall, John's younger brother, Albert, was diagnosed with an incurable, inoperable brain tumor. John was devastated and worried about how Silvia would react. She understood that Albert was gravely ill but repeated that since "they sent him home from the hospital, the doctors must not be worried." I was edgy, as John was once again thrown into the middle of family crises, this time on two fronts. He distracted himself with St. Louis's winning football and baseball teams. I stayed active in my church, where worship brought me solace. I wrote in my old people's journal. Yet, like those at sea, we were in peril as we waited for Albert's and Silvia's diseases to play out. I felt helpless.

Silvia fell two times within thirty-six hours on the first weekend of December. Both times she used her Lifeline to bring help. "Lifeline" is a device worn as a bracelet or a necklace that, when its button is pushed, activates a central "personal response service," manned around the clock for emergencies, especially medical ones. The response monitor "assesses the situation and summons appropriate help" (Lifeline Systems, Inc.). For Silvia and my mother, John and I were designated by Lifeline as the appropriate persons to call for help if an ambulance were not needed.

Like a recipe code, a Lifeline is useful—as long as its owner wears it and remembers how to use it. On her second fall, Silvia smashed her left wrist, requiring surgery with pins to fix it and a daunting metal apparatus on her forearm. Silvia did not activate her Lifeline after either December fall. She somehow crawled or hoisted herself up; then she waited for Sandra to arrive.

9

The Sweet Survival Dogwood Tree
2001

January capped a series of terrible months—so terrible that my woe-mometer rose to ten. Around me, close friends were dealing with demanding end-of-life situations. Helen and Mark watched over his older Parkinson's-ridden brother, while Richard and Roz coped with his nonagenarian folks in New York City. Jack and Lillian were occupied with their two frail mothers. Then John was diagnosed with a ruptured floating disc in his lower back. The pain radiating down his leg was so intense that he was only comfortable sitting. He could not walk. It was as if all the anxiety of his parents' and brother's illnesses spawned severe back problems that made him uncomfortable in almost any position. An orthopedic surgeon would operate on him in early February.

As the New Year began, we hired around-the-clock care for Silvia. Sandra, her regular caregiver, was the mainstay of the team. Because one of Silvia's hearing aids was broken and because of her growing confusion, she was a challenging patient. A nurse's aide who loved plants asked Silvia how she took care of her plants. Silvia reacted angrily: "Don't ever ask me to give you my pants!"

Silvia's apartment in her senior residence abounded with impressive plants, tall and glossy green. Silvia had grown two or three of the plants from seedlings she purchased at a supermarket. They thrived for decades on the tiled sun porch off Paul and Silvia's living room. The sun porch afforded perfect growing conditions, with tall windows on three sides, including a southern exposure, where pale winter sunlight poured onto ficus, dracaena, and palm specimens. In ever larger pots, plants framed low bookcases and gave the sunroom a greenhouse atmosphere in the dead of winter.

Silvia coddled her plants. She used a moisture-measuring gadget; she repotted plants when white tendrils of the roots threaded out the drain holes into the saucers; she dusted and polished the leaves. Each spring she and Paul used a dolly to wheel the plants to the swimming pool deck. There they passed the summer like sentinels watching over the pool's blue water and bobbing toys, the tumble of geraniums and impatiens, basil and Italian parsley in surrounding garden beds.

When Silvia decided she could not live alone in the big house if Paul were placed in a nursing home, she and John had selected an apartment in the independent living section of a retirement center. The apartment's balcony was perfect for two chairs, a small table, and Silvia's plants, which she moved with her. The balcony and the year-round sunlight allowed the plants' inside-outside routine to continue. Silvia used myriad products to fend off whiteflies and encourage miracle growth, and she misted the leaves when dry winter heat threatened them.

Silvia was as sensitive to the deadness of winter as the flowers she tended. When January's sunlight turned watery, Silvia needed lively, vivid color. On trips to the supermarket with Sandra, Silvia always fell for a blooming plant—an African violet, a cyclamen, or an azalea in the deepest of reds. One winter day when I arrived at her apartment, she said, "Susan, have you seen this wonderful kalanchoe with all its little yellow flowers? It looks bright these winter days, doesn't it?" She turned its tiny yellow flowers with red centers up toward me, as if introducing a new face.

Silvia tired, too, of winter's dark clothes, and she would never wear black. In her closets full of clothing collected over her American lifetime, there was not a single black cocktail dress among the fuchsia, purple, and magenta silk dresses. The rainbow array of cotton jersey polo shirts she favored for yard work harbored not one black top. Her skirts and suits were navy, aubergine, claret, charcoal gray, with taupe or beige for warm months, but never black. Her lingerie, some in silk and satin from Italy, lay folded in shades of peach or blush pink or ivory. Paul, I learned, preferred she not wear black because it reminded him of fascism. The slacks in her residence closet were all new purchases acquired after Paul's death, for he also disliked her wearing trousers.

In her apartment, without responsibility for a pool or a garden, Silvia spent hours every day caring for her plants. She had planted the yard of the St. Louis house on Overhill Drive, where she and Paul lived for forty years, with beds of hostas, ground cover, and flowering shrubs like rhododendron. The swimming pool nestled into a slender side yard. One year, she tried arugula as a border plant; another season, she planted a giant hollyhock-like perennial that she found ungainly but couldn't bring herself to pull out; she tucked impatiens in ivy beds and basil wherever she found an empty spot. But Silvia's masterpiece, planted beside the house on the swimming pool's border, was a Japanese-like pink dogwood tree, curved asymmetrically and set in an oval space next to the fence, where it provided a bit of shade at the sunny east end of the pool.

One winter, a vicious ice storm destroyed or deformed many trees in

St. Louis. Outside her dining room doors, Silvia saw the pink dogwood tree—many of its branches had snapped and fallen onto the winter pool cover. Other branches dangled, with only the trunk and one or two substantial limbs intact.

"What shall I do?" she asked at Sunday lunch, as we looked out at the skeleton of the dogwood and the grotesque, glistening debris.

"Nothing to do. It's ruined."

"Cut your losses. Chop it down."

"Plant a new tree in spring."

"Ice storms are killers. The tree will never come back."

We were all doomsayers.

"When the ice melts, I'll get out there and clean up the mess," Silvia said. "I have good pruning shears. I can trim the tree back. I'll see what happens."

Silvia looked at her broken dogwood as she looked at the world: I can make this tree revive. I can be of help. I, on my own, can make a small difference.

The pink dogwood came back to life. Silvia's eye for design and her strong pruning hands shaped a smaller tree, compact in shape, steady in its rebirth, and ready to bloom its four-petaled pink blossoms again in a few years. I thought of this tree as her "sweet survival dogwood"—its beauty and perseverance reflective of Silvia's nature.

—◊—

On a cold February day, I visited my mother. When she didn't answer the doorbell, I peered into the living room window. Her head bent over a book, she wore thick glasses and held the book close to her eyes. I saw how well-dressed she was: soft sweater trimmed with fabric matching her green-brown tweed skirt. She sat in a flowered armchair close to a lighted fire, surrounded by old family furniture; books she loved, including a volume of a French *Book of Hours*; and the crystal dish filled with chocolate. YumYum, her Siamese cat, sat curled on her lap.

I knocked on the door, tried the handle. The door opened.

"Mom, it's me."

"Oh dear." She was startled. "Susan? I must have dozed off."

"Do you feel okay?" I pulled a chair close to her.

"Yes. Why?"

"I worried when you didn't answer."

"Bored. I'd have to say I'm bored. It's a slow time of year," she said.

"How's the book you're reading?"

"I've had enough of it. There are no books that really interest me right now."

I looked around the living room shelves full of books categorized and alphabetized by my father—reminders of my parents' tastes—*The Forsyte Saga*, Joseph Conrad, E. M. Forster, John O'Hara. My father's political books, war histories, and mountaineering collection lived in the first floor study, while on the second floor, each of the bedrooms held more recent acquisitions and college books Missy, George, and I had abandoned. No, I would not ask my mom whether there wasn't a single book around the house that would catch her fancy.

"How's everything otherwise? It's a tough month—Dad's birthday and the first anniversary of his death."

"I'm lonely. There's not any reason to get dressed. I didn't bother yesterday or the day before."

"Let me go make us some tea. Has Judy baked recently?" Judy kept my mother's sweet tooth satisfied.

"I'd like a piece of that cake she made. I wish Judy were here longer each day."

In the kitchen I prepared the sugar bowl dedicated to afternoon tea.

Mom prescribed sugar cubes and tongs, as well as real cream in a matching pitcher—quaint touches, emblems of my mother for me. I brought the tea with all of its accoutrements, Mom's favorite teacups and saucers, and cake on her cherished tole tray, the handiwork of Mom's sister Mamie, who had died more than forty years ago.

"You know, Mom, you do need more help or more company," I said, as I poured tea for her. I tried to be gentle.

"My friends are so old that they're not very interesting."

"Could you organize anything like lunch with one of them? It would get you out."

"Oh," she sighed. "I just don't know." She ate her cake, balancing the plate over Yummy, asleep in her lap. She had gained twenty pounds in the previous five years, so that she was a stout 165 pounds. The extra weight on what was now a 5'5" frame exacerbated her knee problems, uncured by knee replacement surgery. I had difficulty boosting her into my car for outings.

"Do you want me to look into having Judy work longer hours?"

"Judy annoys me. She's nosey, and she answers the phone before I get there." Mom looked into the fire. "Yes, you could see if she has more hours available for me."

I took this as acquiescence, understanding how our aging parents often presented both sides of an argument as their own before a stance became clear. I asked Judy if she would add hours to her work schedule, although I was uncertain about whether my siblings would accept an added expenditure. Yet, if this were the beginning of our mother's slow fade, then I was determined to create a safe setting that might alleviate her melancholy. That winter, I was lucky to have my teaching to keep me from sinking into a morass of worry about Mom. Classes distracted me from winter's gloom, and John's rest and physical therapy were slowly helping him recuperate from back surgery.

—⁓—

In February 2001, a year after my dad's death, I began a session of the Voyages and Discoveries French literature class with, "Let's hear some reaction to Flaubert's main character, Emma."

Ty shot his arm up, his body levitating from his seat in the front row of the class.

"Emma Bovary sucks!" he yelled.

Laughter burst out from twenty-five students. They snickered because rascal-handsome Ty was the leader of the "way cool" students. He, like most of the students, sensed my awe and reverence for *Madame Bovary*, even though I tried to treat all the works in the course to an evenhanded reading.

I loved these students, loved this fifteen-year-old course of my invention. I had marketed it first to our skeptical department, the majority of whom didn't believe in teaching French works in English. I loved the hard work of winning over these cynical students—chemistry majors, fraternity boys, economics majors, and pre-med seniors fulfilling this final, "Oh-my-God-old-French-books" humanities requirement in their last semester. My challenge was to draw them into the web of French novels and watch them become emotionally and intellectually involved. I marveled when, after four weeks, they could dissect a paragraph from Balzac in the way that French students learn to pull apart texts: words, images, syntax and verb tenses, vocabulary, cadences and sonority, metaphors and symbols. I watched with amazement as they dived into Gide, living his protagonist's voyages to North Africa, then to France, and back to North Africa.

The way the male students sloped back into those molded plastic chairs with their legs stretched out, as if to trip me, didn't faze me. I paced and taught, turned to the window to reflect, questioned, leaned over a dozing student, paced some more, alighted at the board to write a list of the students' comments. Some of the women students, even in this twenty-first century, would cast their eyes down, as if to hide their literary sensibilities behind an invisible veil. The middle-ground students forgot to bring their texts or drifted, but just for a moment, and yet they carefully copied down my words and those of their fellow students transcribed on the board. I loved to entice these young people into the joys of reading a novel from what seemed a faraway place, to convince them that these stories could be their stories, could speak like voices next door of experiences they, in their mere two decades, had experienced themselves. Each of my students, I imagined, had fallen in and out of love, had witnessed an illness close in, and had looked for a way to escape, as had Emma Bovary, Gide's Michel, and Colette's vagabond. These students were my partners in delight for a fleeting semester. I didn't care how they came to the pleasure. Legs stretched out, sloppy notebooks, timid voices or loud, they only needed to follow me until they were ready to take over the helm and captain the journey themselves.

Ty initiated one of those classes in bleak February, when the students came on deck and did the hard work of analyzing that sometimes distant and unattainable heroine, Emma Bovary.

"I wonder," I started slowly as the laughter died away, "if any of you could be more concrete about Emma's evolution in Part II, give us some page citations that we could analyze."

Heads dropped, pages flipped, water was sipped. I loved the silence of students working. It never frightened me or demanded that I fill it. Then crash, cacophony burst on the room.

"Like when she refuses to kiss Leon good bye—that sucks."

"Yeah, so why doesn't she kiss him? She's a tease. I hate that. Like when she and Leon walk out to visit her baby."

"Man, right away she switches from Leon to Rodolphe."

"Rodolphe's just a player, like when he talks about his seduction strategies. She's stupid."

"No, she isn't. She just wants thrills. Do you blame her?"

"Who's talking about blame?"

"Dude, I know someone just like that—calculating with her eyes like Emma at the agricultural fair."

"Please put your page numbers on the board and a two-word reason for why your passage defines Emma."

Winter boots tramped to the board, chalk squeaked, texts opened to underlined passages, outbursts, chatter—the tale of a mid-nineteenth century French provincial adulteress had conquered my class. Nothing, almost nothing felt as good to me. Maybe my grandson's hug or summer naps with John in Pentwater or an over-the-kitchen-counter talk with one of my children, now more than equal adults. A class like this, when the students' energy and insights made learning a joy for all of us, ranked high on my pleasure scale.

—⁂—

An unexpected inner voice had pushed me several years before to tell my department chair that I would retire at the end of the 2000–2001 academic year. That voice announcing my retirement surprised even me. It rose from so deep inside that I couldn't answer friends who asked, why at this moment? Why so long before normal retirement age? It was time for someone new to come on board. I was leaving because I had vowed that I wanted to be at my best teaching self when I set out on my next voyage. I was leaving for new adventures. I was leaving because the call of family beckoned. Three more grandchildren would be born in late 2001. Although the old fathers, Paul and George, were gone, the two mothers, Silvia and Dorothy, called—not a siren call from shores faraway, but a call from the core of myself. Silvia had already departed to a mental land where she did not know whether I still taught. Mom would know and take advantage of my independence as soon as I retired.

I heard myself say to the department chair, "Please begin a search to replace me, but please don't cancel my Voyages and Discoveries course." Please, please let it continue, I thought, because I have discovered so much of myself, so much about young people, so much, semester after semester in those timeless tales: *The Immoralist, The Vagabond, The Stranger,* and *The Lover.* Please hold on to that course in memory of me.

"Thank you, Ty, for getting us started today." Thank you, all of my students.

—⁂—

On Good Friday, April 13, 2001, Mom groomed herself with extra care because Betsy was coming from New York City to be her houseguest. Pretty, with her full face still smooth for her 89 years, Mom had had her hair waved at the beauty salon, her nails polished shell-pink. She dressed in a bright cobalt-blue suit for a drive with Betsy. With her cane and Betsy on one side, Judy on the other side, Mom began to walk down the three brick steps from the back of her house. She fell. In spite of bloody scrapes on her shin that Betsy and Judy covered with bandages, Mom's weekend wasn't marred. Betsy brought magical energy to my parents' home, where she had visited many times. Mom loved Betsy for the memories the two shared of Betsy's mother, Elizabeth the decorator, who created the mustard yellow master bedroom with leafy metal lamps. Cats, too—ancient Egyptian cats, cats on postcards, cats in musicals and poetry, cats remembered from Betsy's family fifty years before—danced through Mom and Betsy's conversations. Betsy's short, wavy brown hair with only a hint of gray emphasized her tall, lithe figure. She usually wore jeans and a simple dark sweater. Her dress and athletic figure made her seem ageless, although on this Easter weekend visit she was at least 65 years old. Betsy treated my mother as if she, too, were ageless. She swept Mom off on excursions to revisit the St. Louis where Betsy had grown up before going away to school, a teaching job, then a publishing position. In retirement, Betsy had committed herself to becoming an artist. One acquaintance had invited Betsy to work at a studio in Belize. Another offered her a cottage in Scotland, where Betsy's only duty was to ride the horses.

Betsy arrived in St. Louis with a sack of books for Mom. She presented works on India, a treatise on global poverty, and the latest work by a controversial, internationally famous scholar. Each book touched the connection between Mom and Betsy: the cats they loved, global issues for women, pictures of places one or the other had visited. So enchanted with Betsy's visit was Mom that she didn't notice her skinned legs during the entire weekend.

On April 24, 2001, John's brother, Albert—with Silvia's craggy features and bushy hair like an Afro; who throughout his adult life helped other people: volunteering with VISTA, the domestic peace corps, then nursery school teaching, career counseling, and mentorship of parents adopting children from South America; who ached for anyone hurting—died of a brain tumor at age 54, leaving his wife Lynn and two children, ages 14 and 11. John and I had gone together to visit Albert as soon as John could travel after his back surgery. The day before Albert died, John flew to Washington, D.C., to say good-bye to his brother, and John and I spent the next weekend with Lynn and the children. A few weeks later, we flew out with Silvia for Albert's memorial service.

At Sunday lunch the week after Albert's service, Silvia seemed vacant except when it came to Albert's death. She was 100-percent aware that he had died and asked, "Why couldn't it have been me?"

—◊—

I retired after twenty-four years of university teaching in June 2001.

In Pentwater that July, I relaxed and cleared my head. I reread Dickens's *Great Expectations* and a literary offshoot called *Ahab's Wife* by Sena Jeter Naslund, which almost pushed me to reread *Moby Dick*, but not quite. Our daughter Carol and her husband Noel visited; Carol was five months pregnant with their first baby. As tall as I, she looked long and athletic; her belly barely peeked out from a tankini-type swimsuit. I gave a baby shower for her. While Noel—ruggedly good-looking, steady, quiet, and thoughtful—drove north to fly-fish a trout stream and John played tennis, Carol and I mixed blueberries into muffin batter and sliced strawberries for the shower. She was as organized and competent in the kitchen as in her education policy job. Her movements were quick, graceful, natural, as she worked from a sixth sense about combinations of ingredients and quantities, especially for baked goods.

I invited our lifelong summer friends—Shirley, a lively widow who walked 3 miles north and back on the beach each afternoon; her granddaughters Maddy and Beth; and Ruth, a crack golfer who knew every bird in our Michigan forest. They presented miniature blue jeans and a tiny cap, bibs, and a bear with a tinkling bell inside for the new baby.

That night, as we sat on the porch watching the sun set, then spread flat across the horizon and turn from orange to violet to a lingering strip of yellow, Carol mused, "I wonder if the time has come to have a family parade tomorrow night. Noel has never been to one."

Before I could answer, before John said anything, before the dark night sky swallowed all color, Carol answered herself: "It is too soon."

Too soon after Dad's death, after the summers of the 1980s and 1990s, when we gathered, so many of us, including Will's high school football buddies, the women in Carol's high school Awesome Eightsome group, and Ellen's friends—too soon to imagine how we might recompose ourselves as a family, to explain to each other without embarrassment that we would continue to celebrate one another with parades, to cling together in hard times, to rejoice in the chain of my Coleman grandparents aunts uncles parents cousins siblings, waving an old flag, beating pots in a procession on a beach strewn with silvery driftwood and seagull droppings and zebra mussel shells, on a beach long enough to stretch the chain of our family on these white sands back more than seventy-five years.

I was relaxed in Pentwater that July because I no longer juggled so many things. The academic year 2000–2001 had been an emotional roller coaster. I'd retired from teaching and my academic career, where I thrived in the classroom and in mentoring students. I was worn out from dealing with the end of my professional life and John's back surgery, successful as it was; with Albert's death; and with increased mother and mother-in-law care, raising the specter of Alzheimer's disease—theirs and, maybe in the years ahead, our own. I needed that Michigan month to ease the fearful and traumatic prospect that my fate, that John's were foreshadowed by our parents' last days. In the quiet and serenity of Pentwater, I rediscovered my spirit and sense of humor about the wry absurdity of these times.

George, back in St. Louis, phoned and recounted that on Friday, a few days earlier, Mom had fallen in the mud room and summoned help with her Lifeline. Like Silvia, she wore the device around her neck. I wondered whether this fall and her fall on Good Friday when Betsy was visiting were signs of ministrokes or diminished balance. I believed that falls were inevitably serious and symptomatic of something unknown, maybe unknowable. My siblings, however, saw them as old-age commonplaces. At that time, we did not have the benefit of what doctors now know: falls are comparable to strokes in the harm they can do. They require complex,

wide-ranging interventions. Instead, my brother and I agreed that batteries of tests would not be useful. We decided that, Zen-like, we would
wait to see what lay ahead.

In the summer of 2001 Silvia could barely walk or get up from a chair,
although she attended a balance class at her residence. We suspected that
she had fallen more than we knew.

I felt as if death from falling loomed for both mothers. Basically,
Dad had died of a broken hip from a fall, followed by surgery that doctors touted as the only way that he—a rail-thin, arthritic, demented
90-year-old man—would walk again, a surgery that had led to bodily
system breakdowns during his "recuperation." Each time our mothers
fell, I empathized with them, sensing their despair and increasing vul-
nerability.In their phone calls, they sounded pitiful, startled, affronted by
their bodies' failures. Falls rendered them alternatively fearful, stubborn,
compliant, sad, defiant, and resigned. Yet, we thought there was precious
little we could do to stop their falling.

—∞—

The events of September 11, 2001, hung over the country and over
us as a family. About two weeks later John had his first partial seizure,
a frightening few moments in which he stumbled and staggered as we
crossed Delmar Boulevard on our morning walk with Rufus, the basset
hound we adopted soon after Winston died. After all John's caregiving
years as a father, a brother, and a son, all the happenings in his life and in
the world's life, I felt as if his mind and body may have come unhinged
as he sat on the curb, disoriented, not speaking, staring at but not seeing
me. He spent a night in the hospital, his diagnosis unclear. The doctors thought a ministroke was a possibility. Our naïve hope was that

this terrifying episode was an anomaly, something that would never be repeated.

At the end of September, Missy and her husband, Walt, moved to Colorado. They had long dreamed of retirement there. They moved with Labrador retrievers, skis, and the promise of a relaxed, outdoorsy life. I felt a fierce mixture of excitement and admiration for them, of sadness and abandonment, of jealousy and jubilation for a freedom that tempted yet eluded me.

That autumn, the two mothers sapped whatever coping energy I had. The interplay between their crises might have been a sketch from the French Theater of the Absurd. Samuel Beckett, for one, does wicked sketches of aging. At times, I felt as if I were one of Beckett's characters on the plodding, futile march toward death.

After another fall, Mom said, "Don't tell me to use a walker. I was bending over. That's all, bending over to pick up Yummy." I could picture Yummy, her ears laid back, tail a-bristle, fleeing Mom with a mischievous gleam in her eyes.

On the answering machine, a message from Silvia: "My purse is gone. Gone with my checkbook. I buzzed my Lifeline because my hearing aids aren't working."

And Mom next told me: "Tina, that new helper you got me, is no help at all. None. She gives me lunch an hour late because she's carving an apple into a flower for Waldorf salad—if she even gets here in time for lunch. Something about her boyfriend last time."

At Sunday lunch, Silvia looked at John at the head of our dining room table: "Are you John?"

"What do you mean, Mamma?" he asked.

"I think you're my brother. Is there another John?"

"Mamma, I'm John, your son."

"You know, some strange men dropped me off here."

"I brought you here in my car," John spoke slowly, as if he were talking to a child.

Later that autumn, my mother phoned, "I had your brother come over this morning. I didn't want to disturb you so early."

"Why, Mom?"

"Because I fell in the night."

"And your Lifeline?"

"I didn't have it on. After all, it was the middle of the night. I don't need it. It was George's turn."

"Are you okay?"

"Tina's not coming today. She called. Something about her mailbox being knocked down. Cry eye, why wouldn't I be okay? I'm cross at Tina."

After an early morning call from Sandra, John asked her to pass the phone to Silvia: "Mamma, Sandra says your eye is bloodshot and your arm is bruised. Did you fall? Are you all right?"

My mind raced during those early morning hours when every worry, every fear turned into its own worst possible scenario: I'm okay, just fine, checkbook's gone, Lifeline's hanging on the bedpost, doing fine, fell chasing the cat, lost my hearing aids, tumbled over. It's 4 a.m. Perfect, it was my brother's turn. I'm almost crazy with worry about John; he's blind and deaf to me, John, my partner for picnics and music and Michigan. Tests with dye light his brain functions. God, may they show nothing, rien, nada, nothing at all. Oh, for cry eye, my mom's strongest epithet; these falls and lapses and episodes hardly count as crises; don't worry, why should I worry, what good does it do? They're mere pops of trouble that burst like bubbles, fade away, erupt some place else in different colors, 'growing-old flickers,' they're called. I investigate, follow up whenever our moms phone, and I wonder—yes, marvel, how did I hold a job and what happens to old people who have no one to react to or to advocate for them or to intervene to spare them from oblivion? And I wonder what will happen to me, to John. I am afraid.

In November, I fired Tina, Mom's creative, apple-carving but unreliable caregiver, whom I'd hired to keep Mom company on weekends and evenings, as Judy could not work longer hours. I felt embarrassed because Tina had come highly recommended by a close friend. Yet Tina could not keep to a schedule, and her tales of an inattentive boyfriend and a mailbox destroyed in the dark of night filled my mother with anguish. I, too, anguished over Tina's problems and our problems with her, wished we could find someone as wonderful as Dorth, and realized I was not cut out for personnel management.

Donna, the social worker whose expertise and advice we relied upon, took some of the heat off me. Her voice on the phone soothed me, although her charges were substantial. She frequently took Mom out for lunch and shopping, as if they were old friends, yet such outings were an expensive form of therapy. Donna needed, she explained to me, time, slow time, to get an older person like my mom to trust her enough to open up. Donna located another caregiver-housekeeper to assist Mom when Judy wasn't there, and she found a new psychiatrist who prescribed an antidepressant for Mom, something Missy and I thought she'd needed for quite some time. My sister and I both surmised that Dad had lured our mom from past depressions with major excursions, the suggestion of a new civic project, or a party to host. Years ago, Mom had taken an antidepressant and even gone to some talk-therapy sessions. With unusual candor, she'd confessed to her reading group that she had sought help. The women had been startled because such an admission was rare for anyone of their generation. Mom's friends, she reported, admired and supported her. However, after several months, Mom had taken herself off the medication and stopped talk therapy, unbeknownst to Missy or me at the time. Compliance was not Mom's strong point.

During that fall of 2001, the leaves on Paul and Silvia's survival dogwood tree were among the first to turn color, curl, and then drop. If a summer in St. Louis is dry, from the top of a dogwood tree spreading downward, the green leaves lighten in a last burst of photosynthetic energy in September. Then by October they turn a bright orangish-red, announcing the change of seasons. In readiness for its sweet blossoms in spring, the tree sets autumn buds—tight, abundant ones. A surprise wind blows from Canada, sweeps away the golden Missouri Indian summer, and sends the dogwood's now curled leaves in a torrent onto the pool cover and down the driveway at Paul and Silvia's former house. The buds cling to the branches, harbingers of the carefree blooms the dogwood will produce next April, for those buds have no memory of the damaging ice and radical pruning that saved their tree's life. Silvia's valiant tree will burst forth for the new family who bought the house, a family with children whose voices rise in summer from the pool deck as we walk by.

Like the buds of promise on the dogwood, three new lives burst forth in that transformational fall of 2001. John and I would groan when the phone rang after ten at night or before eight in the morning, as we tried to divine which of our mothers the call would be from and whether it would herald what is called in the senior citizen trade "a precipitating crisis." Instead, the phone that autumn became our lifeline, because daughter Carol and daughter-in-law Sara were due to have babies in the fall of 2001. Will and his petite, active, and dancer-graceful wife, Sara, awaited twin girls. Both families now lived in Seattle.

Suddenly the babies came, announced over the phone by our breathless, astonished children, who were now our peers as parents. The twin girls arrived several weeks before their due date; they were healthy and ready to go home from the hospital after three weeks. Will called their baby daughters the "littles."

About six weeks later, in November, along came another "little." Sam was born to Carol and Noel in that frightened, suspended period following September 11, when the glow of autumn felt like an affront, when fear of planes and terror and foreignness and powdery white anthrax made me weep at the slightest contretemps. Sam was born on a day so brilliant that it reminded me of 9/11 and triggered more tears. The sound of fighter planes overhead made my body tense.

While I was in Seattle to help Carol with baby Sam and cheer her on as a new mother, I opened their front door to get the mail one day.

"Don't, Mom. We're leaving the mail outside until Noel gets home. He'll check it to be sure it's safe before he brings it in," Carol said. Terrorism had struck again that fall with mysterious anthrax attacks coming through the mail.

For Thanksgiving in Seattle, John and I prepared a dinner for the two new families with their littles. We shopped in organic food stores, blended our St. Louis ritual with our children's wedding-gift cookware, recipes, and ceremonies. The twin girls celebrated the meal—one strapped to each parent's chest, their blond heads nestled so close that they must have rocked with each adult swallow of turkey or sweet potatoes. Little Sam lay in the curl of Noel's forearm, his perfect bald head rested in his father's bent elbow, so that his two-week-old eyes could watch this expanded family he had joined, as we rejoiced for him and his cousins, for the life that every cry or gassy smile represented in that moment of national terror.

Soon after these babies presented themselves, Ellen with her 2-year-old son, Devon, the oldest grandchild of our expanding family, came to St. Louis for a weekend visit.

I was cooking dinner in the kitchen when Devon handed me a package.

"What's this, Dev?"

"A present for you, Nana."

"For having us here, Mom," Ellen added.

I unwound crumpled tissue paper to find a jar of New England blackberry jam from a farm near Ellen's town in Massachusetts. I love jam. I eat jam from a spoon as a snack when no one's around at midday or on the way to bed after settling Rufus. I once read that Virginia Woolf also ate jam—I believe she favored strawberry—directly from a spoon. After Devon's birth, I vowed to myself that I would instill my deeply held belief in the joys of jam in each grandchild. I would undertake this training privately, once they were old enough, away from their parents, a pleasure to be shared, to be reveled in with Nana alone.

"How did you know, Dev? I love blackberry jam. We'll have it together tomorrow for breakfast," I said.

"One more gift, Mom," Ellen said.

"Wow, Ellen. You didn't need to."

"We're going to have another baby in June."

The downturn of Ellen's deep blue eyes, the soft pride in her voice—her kitchen annunciation to accompany blackberry jam—temporarily erased the fears and instability of that late fall season.

"Another little! Well, El, that's wonderful! What a passel of kids our family will have and yet another for me to train on blackberry jam."

So, in the fall of 2001, the sweet survival dogwood tree lived on. Its leaves spun away into the north wind, announcing winter as the buds silently prepared for spring. For a moment, three new babies eased John's and my angst about his health and our mothers' declines. Ellen's baby would grow through the winter and arrive as the survival dogwood leafed to its fullest, casting shade against the hot St. Louis summer. With the arrival of grandbabies, I began to feel as if I would survive, pruned and reshaped as I might be.

In November, while the United States prepared to attack Afghanistan, I asked Mom if I could borrow Dad's Afghanistan travel file. I wanted to compare the country she and Dad had visited with the country the United States was poised to invade, whose oppressive Taliban government we were set to overthrow.

Eyes narrowed, Mom pointed a finger at me and said, "Don't you lose that file." How could Mom imagine I'd be careless with one of my father's files?

The file was filled with out-of-date facts about Afghanistan's government in the 1970s and picture postcards of ancient cultural artifacts, like a giant Buddha that had been wrecked in a fundamentalist purge of art, one file among hundreds in the old cabinet that somehow hadn't tipped over onto Dad.

In the late fall, Mom's and Silvia's old age paths diverged. The manager of Silvia's residence called to say that she could no longer go to the symphony in a van with the group of fellow residents, as she was too likely to stray, to talk during the concert, or to be incontinent. Soon afterward, the residence staff reported that Silvia wandered the halls all night and had tried to leave by herself "to go downtown for breakfast."

The residence staff was at their collective wit's end and demanded that we hire around-the-clock care for Silvia. And Sandra, her daytime caregiver, had reported rapid changes in Silvia's behavior and cognitive abilities. John decided that Silvia would have to be moved to "assisted living," a higher level of care within the same facility. John had a hard time facing the move. I felt his tension in his crankiness. He couldn't bring himself to believe that his mother had reached this point. John was concerned that Luciana might oppose a move because it would mean Silvia's giving up the apartment and her domestic independence. The alternative—around-the-clock care in her apartment—would substantially increase costs, and temporary caregivers would not provide a consistent routine for Silvia in the evenings and on weekends when Sandra was not there.

Silvia was miserable during the holiday season. She confused John with her brother, couldn't recognize faces in family pictures in her apartment, and told me, "I should have stayed in Italy. There is no one for me here."

To John, she said, "My parents abandoned me. I never saw them except when I was an infant child."

"But, Mamma," John paused. He remembered that the Alzheimer's Association cautions family members and caregivers not to correct or try to straighten out the muddle that patients express.

"I feel lonely and abandoned," Silvia said, "and I don't like having all those different women with me at all hours of the day. I don't know what to talk to them about."

"I'm working on it, Mamma. Working on the systems."

To John, Silvia's words were a clear call for help.

—⁓—

As 2001 ended, my mother's mood lifted. Donna functioned as paid listener, counselor, and companion for outings. She caught on to Mom's taste for luxury, which led the two to shop for extravagances like pink calfskin mules to serve as slippers. Together, Mom and Donna often lunched at a mall where one restaurant's popovers with honey butter delighted Mom so much that she phoned me to rave about them. When Donna was not available, Mom expected George or me to entertain her.

With me, Mom enjoyed preparations for her ninetieth birthday party in March; we made guest lists, selected invitations, and studied menus. George, long-retired, often stopped by to chat with Mom and play with YumYum. Like Mom, he was a cat lover. George and his partner, Gabriele, invited Mom to their home for holidays and family gatherings. On Sundays, John would fetch her to have lunch at our house.

Although Mom could be sharp-tongued about family and acquaintances, she remained loyal to her old friends. She still drove herself to Friday reading group lunches. She went to the theater with Betty and orchestrated the hiring of painters "to spruce up" her house in preparation for houseguests invited to her birthday celebration.

I looked back on 2001 as a year when many of us thought a lot about death. John's brother Albert died in April, and in September almost three thousand people had been killed. Many Americans' belief in our country's indestructibility died then, too. I missed Dad terribly, especially in autumn when I spent time with Mom in the house on Ballas Road, surrounded by the trees Dad had cherished. The cause of John's mysterious seizure was still unknown. We mourned as Silvia's memory and self-confidence faded. And a dynamic part of me had died when I retired from my academic career.

I bumped into death often that year. A colleague quipped that all of French literature is about sex and death. Duras' heroine in *The Lover*, the final book we studied in the Voyages and Discoveries course, repeatedly describes her lovemaking as "pleasure unto death." Death was present all spring in the literature I taught and in memories of the literature I know deeply.

During my last semester of teaching, Emma Bovary's death had filled several days of my life. After describing Emma's final agony from arsenic poisoning, Flaubert, with a stroke of ingenious brevity, pronounces her dead, using the verb "to exist" rather than "to be": "Elle n'existait plus." (She no longer existed.) Despite her shortcomings, Emma had fully existed; she did not languish by the fireside, feeling sorry for herself. My students, many of whom had never met death face to face, squirmed and protested through Emma's death chapter, then breathed more easily when she ceased to exist.

Camus' narrator, Meursault, in *The Stranger* figured later in the course. He cannot, from the first page, get straight in his mind the exact day when his mother died. Today, yesterday, who cares? A mother dead on the first page: that's the stuff of a story. My students discovered in Camus' pages that you're expected to pay attention to your mother's dying and to your actions afterward.

"But it's not fair to judge Meursault."

"He's just being honest."

"So what if he goes to a comic movie right after his mom dies?"

"And sleeps with his girlfriend."

"He has the right."

"He's just honest."

Yes, his mother was so old that Meursault had felt obliged to send her to a nursing home. Who has the right to criticize his apparent lack of grief? At least, though, we expect him to feel a little guilt or sorrow.

In April 2001, I had written each student in the Voyages and Discoveries course a letter of thanks for his or her acute insights as we'd journeyed through books I'd come to inhabit as closely as if they were my skin.

When my academic days were over, death haunted me in the visual terrors of September eleventh, the harsh scenes splashed repeatedly on TV screens and narrated by solemn broadcasters. In the autumn of 2001, death had lost the simplicity of Charles Bovary's passing, tightly written by Flaubert. My psyche could not comprehend September's horrendous deaths.

I caught myself muttering, "Hurry up please it's time" from T. S. Eliot's "The Waste Land" after a visit to my mother on a late November afternoon. Mom's moods had grown less predictable. Though I told myself I wasn't responsible for her happiness, her sadness that day overwhelmed me. Back at home, after the umpteenth lost-purse call from Silvia, thinking of each mother, I said, "Oh, please do hurry up with this dying business. Hurry up please it's time." Zap, bang.

And as I murmured Eliot's lines, guilt gnawed at me.

Then came life—lots of it, fresh, squalling, burping, right into my heart, right into the heart of our family. Whenever I think about Silvia's certain vision and strong hands that resurrected the pink dogwood tree, I remember to focus on life.

10

A Helmet in the Attic
2002

Silvia's move to the assisted living quarters proved timely. In the first months of the year, she had a vacant look, her once lively eyes now flat, dark pools. She gained weight in her new environment, where she ate meals in a communal dining room. She became incontinent, which limited outings except to the doctor. She inquired politely about where I lived, but we could no longer bring her to our house for Sunday lunch because any change from her familiar environment confused her. Thanks to Bingo games, her dining mates, and her room, which John arranged to mimic her old house and previous apartment, Silvia seemed well cared for.

In her new room, John hung vintage photos of Paul and Silvia, both looking like 1930s' movie stars. The tilt of the head, the suave flat waves of hair, and the mischief in their eyes made the pictures alluring, even seductive. Silvia must have looked like this when Paul courted her. Silvia identified the photo of her young self, noting shyly how "pretty" she was.

After Silvia's move to the assisted living wing, John could not at first bring himself to visit her. His mother's pared-down existence and her narrow range of responses—"Hello, are you really John?" or "Hello, are you my brother?"—stabbed at John and often kept him away for days.

—⁓—

On March 4, 2002, Missy, George, and I held a cocktail party for our mother's ninetieth birthday. I had coached Mom as she made lists during the winter months. We shopped together for invitations, and she addressed the envelopes. She and I met to sample hors d'oeuvres at the club where the party would be held. We ordered flowers. She kept a tally by her phone of 'yes' and 'no' responses. About thirty friends and relatives accepted the invitation. Betsy, her book- and cat-loving friend, came to stay in Mom's freshly painted house. Cousin Lanny, Mom's nephew and son of her late sister Mamie, flew in from Boston. Donna and her husband attended. Donna introduced herself to many of the women she'd heard about from Mom during their shopping and lunch outings and gave her card to several. The entire reading group came to the party. None of our children could be there because of infants and jobs, although Missy's daughters, Molly and Anna, added youthfulness to the festivities.

Mom wore a new silk dress with a swirling, Chinese pattern in teal and aquamarine and fashionable, low-heeled pumps. Her reading group friends also wore silk print dresses in bright colors, their white hair carefully groomed in waves. Faith Amos wore her signature black hat, wide brim shading her eyes, as she steadied her husband on his non-cane side.

On the evening of the party, the club room glowed with dimmed lights. Outside the vast windows, St. Louis buildings and cars' headlights twinkled. Mom stationed herself next to a wingback chair, an arrangement of roses on a table next to her. She could lean on the chair or sit in it if she tired—a stage set she planned in advance. The excitement as she greeted friends flushed her face. I stood nearby and offered her a glass of wine. She seemed almost breathless as she singled out each guest:

"Betty, dearie, can you believe we're here, right here together in our nineties now?" Mom said to Betty T., whose veined hand she held.

"Oh, Maude," she greeted one of Dad's cousins, "Wouldn't George have loved this party and all these wonderful people?"

A server brought a microphone to the center of the room. Mom's friends settled on couches and straight chairs, stashing walkers and canes out of the way. Several nibbled at the peanuts Mom had ordered for the side tables, reminiscent of parties at her home. The toasts began: Missy, George, and I; one of Mom's granddaughters; a rhyming ditty by Patricia; and remembrances and admiration from Betty T. Finally, Mom, whose voice did not project as well as it used to, full of emotion, spoke. Her face shone softly; her words of thanks were clear to friends and relatives.

Late that night, John, Lanny, Missy and her husband, Walt, and I sat around our fire, reveling in the party and Mom at 90.

Lanny, whose mother, Aunt Mamie, had died of an embolism in her late forties, asked,

"Has your mother, like my mother, suffered from depression all her life?"

"Sorry, can't tackle that tonight, Lanny," I said. "Let's talk about it some other time after the celebration's over." In the midst of all the caregiving for our mothers and worry about John's mysterious ailment, I could scarcely define my own or John's condition. Certainly not my mother's: maybe she'd inherited the tendency toward depression, or was her numbness a result of the interminable, downward spiral into old, old age? I couldn't face such a discussion that evening.

Eight days after the party, Judy called me in the morning.

"Your mother's pulse is 38," she said. "I don't think that's normal."

I was in too much of a hurry to ask what had led Judy to check Mom's pulse. "Call her doctor right away, okay? Tell him everything you observe. And let me know."

Minutes later, Judy called back to say that I was to meet her and Mom at a nearby emergency room. The day's events raced by. At the end of it, after Mom's ambulance transfer to a second hospital and an operation to implant a pacemaker, George and I gasped when the cardiac surgeon said,

"Your mother's doing fine. However, she had a close one. She had no heart function at all for twelve seconds before the implant. Twelve seconds on the other side."

"On the other side?" I asked. "Now what?"

"We'll have her home in a couple of days. She'll need a lot of care."

Several days after Mom went home, Donna talked to her about the options: around-the-clock care at home or temporary placement in a nursing facility until we could ascertain how her heart function was. Mom chose the latter, and Donna selected Villa Manor Assisted Living, where Mom would have a large single room with a bay window, overlooking a grassy lawn and Bradford pear trees. I moved her on March 22. She was 90 years old plus eighteen days. She seemed tired and faint. She slurred her words. But her spirit surfaced when she asked me how her friends could find her to thank her for the wonderful cocktail party.

Judy went daily to Mom's house to bring in mail, switch lights on and off, check phone messages, and feed and soothe YumYum, whom Mom missed fiercely.

In early April, I negotiated with the administration at Villa Manor to allow YumYum to move into Mom's room with her. The litter box would be kept in the adjoining bathroom and dry cat chow in a covered bin. The supervisor required a $200 deposit against cat damage. Yummy's move to Villa Manor with her catnip toys and kitty treats signaled that my mother would stay on in the assisted living facility. After the pacemaker operation, Mom needed carefully monitored medications and on-call assistance. She had never been compliant in following a medication regimen; this was cause enough to require a nursing home, which was much less expensive than round-the-clock care plus housekeeping at home. She would eat three meals a day in the dining room. A nurse's aide would distribute and monitor her extensive medications, including several new ones to control blood pressure. Some she had ostensibly taken for a number of years—a thyroid regulator and an antidepressant. She would use a walker and receive physical therapy twice a week to help her avoid falling.

When YumYum and I arrived in Mom's room, she said, "I could weep tears of joy." And she hugged Yummy in her arms.

What an April! John had another episode, still unidentified. He stumbled in the bathroom, lurched against the sink, became incoherent, then blank, and remembered nothing of those moments, including a phone call he made to our pharmacy. The episode led doctors to perform more heart and brain tests—all inconclusive. John's and my stress and fear levels were magnified by not knowing what had caused the two spells.

One spring day Sandra called to tell us that Silvia had indicated in gestures that she had hidden her new hearing aids in her vagina. I gasped, "What?" I couldn't believe it. Nothing had ever prepared me for this. John and I felt as if we were living in an alternative universe or on the set of a Theater of the Absurd play. X-rays two days later showed no sign of the hearing aids. We imagined that she may have intended to hide them in the bathroom but had accidentally flushed them down the toilet. Without hearing aids, Silvia was more isolated, more turned in on herself, and seldom used spoken language at all.

When I visited Silvia later that week, a supervising nurse in her unit began a chat with me: "Silvia's doing okay mentally."

"What do you mean?" I asked as politely as I could.

"Well, the nurses report that she's quite verbal."

"What could they mean?" I thought about how rarely Silvia spoke.

"They even tell me," continued the official, "she talks in another language really well. In fact, mostly she speaks that language. She's an intelligent woman."

"Excuse me," I bought time to compose myself. "Excuse me, do they know what she's saying or what language it is? Have they ever heard her speak English?"

I wondered whether anyone had looked at her chart for her place of birth. Someone must have noticed the old map of Italy, the photos and etchings of Venice in her room. What about an accent when she does speak English? Please, if this home is truly for Silvia's care, please prepare yourselves with basic information about her.

"Oh well," the official said, "sometimes she repeats one word a lot: 'you-toe' or something like that."

"Could it be 'aiuto'"?

"Probably. She says it a lot, plus an 'aeey' sound I'm not familiar with."

"'Aiuto' means 'help.' Please help." I tried to be calm. "It's Italian, her mother tongue. She's nearly lost her English. And the 'aeey' sound is the way Italians say 'ow' or 'ouch.' She hurts; Silvia hurts."

Silvia hurts. Please help her, and please know that she is calling for help in her first language. That's all she can muster, I thought.

But I couldn't say that because I wanted to stand up for my mother-in-law, keep the nursing staff thinking that yes, this once-elegant Venetian lady still had at her fingertips the magic of another language. I didn't want them to know that she had reverted to primitive cries of anguish. Maybe I could save myself, too, from admitting Silvia's condition. For a language person like me, her loss of words, names, and verbal power meant a loss of identity. I needed to cling to the illusion of Silvia as an intelligent speaker of multiple languages. At that moment, I longed for no more upsets, needed relief from the endless worries and stress—John's undiagnosed spells, Silvia's primitive cries for help, my mother's forlorn clutch of YumYum—just so that I could function day by day. Denial? Oh yes, I desperately wanted to switch off a part of my psyche, but I could not. Each mother was too wracked by pain or anxiety or loneliness.

We had hallway encounters with the nursing staff at Silvia's home, plus formal, ritualized "Care Plan" meetings, the trade name for quarterly meetings required by Missouri state law. The cast of characters at meetings appeared to be set in stone: director of nursing, director of nutrition, director of physical therapy, director of recreational activities (such as Bingo, Santa Claus's visit, a pianist-guitarist duo), director of social work, administrative director of the unit, and the unit's head nurse. That made seven of them, as opposed to three of us: John, Sandra, and me. After Silvia's move to the assisted living unit, we had asked Sandra to continue as private-duty caregiver during weekdays. Each of the seven staff members wore paging-buzzing-alerting devices: BlackBerries or PDAs or cellular pagers or vibrating phones or beepers or buds in their ears. They needed to keep track of time because Care Plan meetings at Silvia's facility lasted sixty minutes—one hour only and not a nanosecond longer. After each person played his or her role, the player exited. Like stage prompters, signals went off audibly or inaudibly throughout; they culminated in the blinks, buzzes, and beeps that announced that we had completed the organization of care for our "loved one."

Fred, director of nutrition, began talking after we signed the attendance log.

"Now," he was earnest, "your mother loves her desserts. Those cakes—she often asks for seconds."

John scowled as he scribbled on a yellow legal pad, flipping the pages as he attempted to write verbatim what we heard during those 3,600 seconds.

Sandra tipped her head. "Silvia has gained a bit of weight."

Fred looked startled and flushed, "Well, I don't think so."

"No. She has not," Head Nurse Rose pronounced. She was a broad, fair-skinned, former military nurse. "We weigh weekly. State law."

Sandra added, "Her clothes fit tighter."

Claudia, the director of nursing, a glamorous, no-nonsense blonde, stepped in with her New York accent: "Could we have some numbers?"

Fred fidgeted with his clipboard: "Her intake last week, and she does ask for fresh fruit, too. . . ."

"Weight. What's her weight?" Claudia insisted. John wrote. I watched.

"Let's see," Rose said, "142 last Friday."

"And three weeks ago, it was 136," Sandra said, drumming her fingernails on the conference table. "Isn't that gaining?"

"No. Not really. It's normal."

John pushed his glasses to the bottom of his nose and eyed everyone. "My math tells me that's a weight gain. Now that my mother is nearly immobile, she doesn't need to eat so much. Why do you give her extra cake?"

The director of social work raised her hand like a schoolgirl asking permission to speak: "Because everyone else is having more. Our goal is for her to feel part of the group."

Claudia cleared her throat and stood up, a teacher to her class. She tapped on a laminated document on the wall: "Patients' Bill of Rights. See that? We're required by law to give her the food she wants."

With a nod, Fred seconded Claudia.

John intervened: "I won't have her gaining weight by eating cake, definitely not extra cake."

I felt like pinching myself. I didn't recognize myself as I sat without speaking in that meeting room. I had considered myself a lively sixty-something, retired French teacher who loved to read Flaubert and to hike in the Ozark woods; wife to a handsome man; mother, grandmother, and friend; dog walker and lentil soup chef. That self had disappeared. Instead, my hair was gray, I might need a sleeping pill at night, and I felt the opposite of lively—dreary and worn down. And my dashing husband was alternately worn out or on edge; John's mysterious blank spells may have been his body's way of offering necessary protection. The window-less room, the cast of personnel characters, the time constraints, John's incessant writing, Sandra's long nails tapping the conference table—all drained me of my self and left me almost as blank as John had been in the midst of a spell.

At the meeting, I imagined John ready to launch into the our-family-never-eats-dessert explanation. When we began our marriage, John proclaimed "Italians don't eat dessert, only fruit." And surely not airy, fluffy American cakes, split into multilayers with buttery, sugary icings that John professed never to touch.

In my solid Midwestern family when Dorth ruled the kitchen, we ate dessert every single night of the week. George, Missy, and I could conjure up the tastes: burnt sugar cake with seven-minute boiled icing, milk cake with homemade dark chocolate sauce, floating island, apple pie—"without the cheese is like a kiss without the squeeze"—Dad's mantra each time an apple pie arrived at the autumn table, chess pie (some called it 'jes' pie because of its humble ingredients: cornmeal, vinegar, sugar, butter, and eggs), lemon meringue pie, and coconut cream pie, my favorite. Following my new husband, I forsook dessert in 1965. I arranged artful displays of oranges, pears, and bananas, with grapes draped languidly among them, and ornate Italian grape shears beside them. John and I ate fruit. Yet, as I had noticed Paul doing after Sunday lunch, John had begun to scrounge in the back of a kitchen cabinet. He pulled out a piece of my baker's chocolate. Later he provided his own stash of sweets—chocolate bars or crunchy hazelnut cookies from an Italian bakery. Just a few sweets, not dessert.

Over the years, I lost my taste for nightly sweet desserts, but in restaurants, John would order dessert with a jolly, "I don't get this at home," as he tackled Key lime pie or crème brûlée. We had reversed our dessert roles.

Maybe Silvia, too, harbored a desire to burst loose from the no-desserts credo. John repeated: "This is my mother. No extra desserts."

Fred was beeped, excused himself, departed backstage.

It was the physical therapist's turn: "Silvia comes to therapy three times a week. She just sits in her wheelchair."

Claudia said: "What's the prescription for this?"

"To try to keep her walking."

John went back to writing.

The administrator tuned in: "Is this Medicare covered?"

John was alert again: "By any chance, are we paying privately?"

"You must be, because she can't walk at all and isn't making any progress, so Medicare doesn't cover it."

Sandra looked at me and rolled her eyes. Three times a week, Sandra wheeled Silvia to physical therapy where she dozed, cried out, "Aiuto," or fingered the fabric of her slacks, at a cost of $25 per visit.

John said, "I'd appreciate your checking the costs and who is expected to pay." He was controlled and professional. Only the jagged handwriting on his legal pad revealed his consternation. The physical therapist slipped out.

On we went—social activities, medications to be tinkered with, adult diapers to be purchased. I looked at my watch—seven minutes to go. I could make boiled icing in that time. My mind wandered. Maybe I would bake myself a birthday cake next month—one with icing like Dorth made; I would set the timer for seven minutes and whisk egg whites and sugar with crushed peppermints until it became perfect for sampling, then spreading on an angel cake. My Nana Coleman had eaten half an angel cake in one sitting on the day she had her fatal stroke.

Claudia's crisp voice interrupted me, "Good meeting. I'll see that all the notes get distributed to staff."

John packed the legal pad in his briefcase.

—⁂—

The spring of 2002 was tense and tough as we tried to understand the cause of John's episodes. I prayed that he would not fail, would not have some terrible disease. As figures throughout the Bible say, I was "sore afraid."

For two months after Mom's move to Villa Manor, George, Missy, and I let our parents' house sit empty. April came; the redbud tree by the garage sprang to life. Dad's favorite lilacs by the gate bloomed wantonly; their branches bumped my car, unleashing the sweet, ancient smell of a new season as I made rounds to check the house. Judy came daily to pick up the mail and to switch lights on and off. That suspended period before we made up our minds to sell the house gave Missy a chance to hold one last celebration on the lawn—an engagement party for daughter Molly and fiancé Jeffrey. After that, Tom, the gardener, pulled weeds from the brick walkway occasionally. The lawn mowers whirred around the lawns weekly, a bit careless in their edging. Inside the empty house, the aura of this being someone's home vanished.

No sounds of bubbling water for winter tea came from the kitchen. The aroma of Judy's poppyseed cake faded. On the hall desk by the entrance, no stacks of books were piled to return to the library or loan to a friend. No basket of tennis balls for serving practice sat by the door. The phone on the desk was silent, its answering machine disconnected. Coffee-table magazines from February, Chinese vases, and tarnished silver ashtrays—relics of dinner parties decades before—sat frozen in place. After checking inside, I often needed to sit down and rest on the screened porch, overpowered by the unfamiliar void.

Once it was clear that our mother needed the nursing supervision of Villa Manor—especially the monitoring of her medications and physical therapy—and could no longer live in her home, we let Judy and Tom go. A mowing service kept the grass cut. We moved the pale-green silk bedroom chaise longue, a tall secretary for Mom's papers, a flowered chintz love seat, and some photos of Dad into her spacious room at Villa Manor. We filled two large closets with her clothing.

One June day I drove Mom to her house to choose some coats and other warm outer wear for winter to keep at Villa Manor. I installed her in a chair at the downstairs hall closet.

"Some good news, Mom, before we go to work."

"What's that?"

"Ellen had her baby. She's fine, and so is he. She named him Simon George."

"That's perfect. Just perfect. I hope they'll call him George," she chuckled, as she ran her finger around the brim of a shabby white tennis hat I'd pulled from the closet. "Do you think a great-grandmother should give up playing tennis?"

"Far be it from me...," I said. I remembered the day ten years before when Mom called to say she'd fallen during a women's doubles game on her own tennis court. In the emergency room, after she'd been diagnosed with a broken wrist and several cracked ribs, she told the doctor: "Just because I'm 80 years old and fell this time, don't tell me to stop playing tennis."

In fact, she never played again, although she threatened to.

In that troubled spring of 2002, I was dispirited and shared not a bit of my mom's momentary spunk.

"So the hats go to Goodwill?" I tossed them in a bag.

"Wait a moment. Not those two straw hats. I love the pink ribbon on that boater. Chandler usually invites me to one of his picnics during opera season. I might need the hats for a *fête champêtre*." Chandler was an old friend who wore bow ties and a seersucker jacket. Like my father-in-law, Paul, he always lowered his lips to a woman's hand in greeting.

"Fine, Mom, just fine." I marveled at my romantic, hat-loving mother, who still dreamed of the next party.

"Now, about my mink coat here."

"Missy thought she could use it out there in Colorado where it's really cold," I said.

"Oh, she did?" Mom straightened herself up. "Well, I need it right here for my winter outings, like cocktail parties and dinner lectures."

Vestiges of the past, I thought. You don't live a cocktail-party life any more. Get real, Mom. Admit your age. But I said nothing, skeptical about her nostalgia yet hopeful that her richly textured days would go on forever.

I pulled out jackets, scarves from Scotland, plastic giveaway rain bonnets from the neighborhood gas station, rubber galoshes with jangly buckles, Dad's old walking sticks, and more tennis paraphernalia until Mom had pronounced on everything—firmly, imperiously, garment after garment, hat after hat. In the end, I knew the provenance of everything in the closet and what my mother wanted me to do with each item. By late afternoon, Mom slumped from revisiting so many decades of her life.

Later in June, George, Missy, and I sold our mom and dad's house to the church next door, including negotiations to avoid the house being torn down for the next three years and to restrict usage of the house out of consideration for neighbors. The sale closing date was set for early August. Missy catalogued the household goods—furniture, mountaineering books, old aluminum cooking utensils, family silver flatware, the baby grand piano, trunks with Marine Corps gear, and carefully collected artwork—much of which we shipped to family members. Some items were destined to be stored, some sold at an estate sale. Old costume jewelry, family photos and newspaper articles, lace from Ireland, and my father and grandmother's exchange of letters went to our basement.

George, in particular, couldn't bring himself to part with our father's travel files and their rusty cabinet. As the permanent in-towner, I agreed to store them at the bottom of our wooden basement stairs, where the files gaped and spilled yellowed newspaper clippings. Soon after the files were moved to our house, I searched them in hopes that Dad would somehow emerge. He did not. The files revealed nothing about the man who had traveled so far. Like a scholar, Dad copied history and statistics from source books as he prepared for each trip. He jotted travel logs of what he saw and the ground he covered, but he didn't explain when or how the fascination of Everest had gripped him, nor what early photo or map beckoned him to the Himalayas. From South Africa he wrote observations of exotic warthogs, gnus, and ostriches. In India, he noted place names, such as Udaipur, Benares, and Jaipur. Dad recorded names of villages and inland seas from the Hebrides and the churches that welcomed travelers along the medieval pilgrimage route to Santiago de Compostela—the travel itself, seeing these sights in so many faraway lands, must have been what intrigued him.

That summer of 2002, I pulled file after file from the cabinet and piled them on a bed, where I rifled them as though a treasure would reveal itself in Germany or Spain or India. I am searching for you, Dad, for your boyhood, when you fancied legendary heroes who traversed Asia and Europe and Africa. I cannot picture you in elementary school, doodling on a scrap of paper as you dream of cargos on the Silk Road, because the father I know is neither distracted nor dreamy. Did you ever resemble those heroes, such as Tamerlane, of outsized courage and vision? Or did your trips wash your lawyerly, everyday life with a sweet, intoxicating liquor I can never taste?

The files I strewed over my bed didn't tell me a story. But, Dad, you loved stories and read Kipling's and Conrad's tales to our children when you came on Sunday Grandpa visits. Your grandkids listened attentively, Dad, and reported that when Mowgli died, your voice caught. You couldn't read on, dropped your eyes. Why did you choose the stories you chose? Where, oh where can I find the "you" who yearned to set foot in the Punjab, who saved the Afghan polo ticket stub—if you don't speak the words to me? I long for those words. You have left me with stories and files of other people's words and your own matter-of-fact notes. I am alone, nearly an old woman myself, among tattered manila folders, lists of towns and cities, the disappointing remains of unexplained voyages.

—⁂—

I began to clean out our parents' house in the summer of 2002, after it was sold in June and before the August closing. When George returned from his customary spring stay in his Tuscany cottage, he became my valiant partner at Mom and Dad's house. Missy would have livened up our work with her funny take on family matters, but she was in Colorado. Before George's return, I decided to work in two-hour segments because my soul, my body, my sentimental being could not endure longer sessions. I found myself worn out, quiet at social events, and less energetic in my daily routines. The summer heat and humidity, the sadness of Dad's death, the heart emergency that led Mom to Villa Manor, Silvia's condition, John's still unexplained medical problem, and the end of our parents' heyday all weighed on me.

After these two-hour purges, I would slump into the driver's seat of my car. No music, no news, no stimuli as I waited for the void within me to refill like a country cistern waiting for rain. Some days the ten-mile trip was sufficient, but sometimes I arrived at home still so empty that I plopped into a chair, Rufus our basset hound by my side. I waited for my self to recover.

I started by emptying the attic. It was best to begin early in the day before the St. Louis heat revved up because the attic's windows—all except two—were nailed shut. Heat was just one of the attic's perils. The beams of the V-shaped roof formed eaves that left the perimeter of the attic space nearly inaccessible. Over the years, Mom and Dad had stuffed old leather valises and flat portfolios with keepsakes, shoeboxes with old letters, and shirt boxes full of Christmas decorations under those eaves. To retrieve them, I needed to duck, kneel, and reach into those low spaces. Time and again I'd stand up to hold an old letter or odd object to the light, and bang, I'd knock my head on a beam.

In the 1960s, when our parents moved into the house, Dad attached a hook by the attic door and hung his olive-drab Marine Corps helmet liner on it to wear for protection from the eaves in the attic. Now, to clean out that space, way into its deepest corners, to sift and process and choose what to do with that trove of our family's history, I wore Dad's helmet liner. Its inner webbing flattened my curly hair. I didn't fasten the chinstrap because its leather had cracked and grown rough after almost sixty years.

With only two windows that would open and summer temperatures on the rise, the attic felt like a steam bath. One June day, sweat began to drip from my face onto woodcuts Dad had collected as a young man: a gnarled tree, a horse against mountains, and an etching of Joseph Conrad by Sir David Muirhead Bone. Apparently, Dad's taste for them had faded or wasn't shared by Mom. Sweat fell onto a manila portfolio of my sister's high school paintings—a swirling blue waterscape, crinkled at the edge—and onto the lids of flat dress boxes from Vandervoort's, Montaldo's, Stix, then Dillard's, each holding a generation of Christmas tree lights: fat, multicolored bulbs that morphed over the decades into miniature twinkly white lights, decorative enough to adorn the lawn in summer.

In spite of decades of marriage and life in this house, my parents weren't pack rats. Theirs was not the detritus of a life stuffed away and forgotten. When they saved things, Dad catalogued, labeled, and articulated the "why" of the save, just as he had done with the travel files. At the center of the attic, where the eaves pointed high over my head, I pulled off the helmet and sat cross-legged between two trunks. A wooden trunk with brass fittings housed blankets. The other was marked FRAY-FOR-UREX, a code from World War II when Dad shipped out to the Pacific with the Marines. It was filled with military gear and camping equipment. The camping gear, with rubberized tarps and a clattery aluminum mess kit, represented one last valiant outdoor adventure. When Mom and Dad were in their sixties, they took a horseback trip in Wyoming or Montana, after which Mom vowed she would never sleep on the ground again.

A few years after Mom and Dad's pack trip, I'd asked, "Dad, could we borrow your mess kit for a float trip?"

"Chickadee," his eyes turned ice blue, "I'm surprised at you for asking."

"Well, I thought . . ." and knew instantly from the stony flash of his eyes that this was the wrong request.

"That is our best gear. Your mother and I. . . ."

I hated hearing my father invoke "we." It compounded the rigidity of his stingy position.

"No, you may not borrow the mess kit."

I had never imagined that I would sit alone, cross-legged in my parents' attic, with power to judge the fate of this tightly guarded treasure.

"Trash," I muttered and pulled a black trash bag close so I could dump Dad's camping treasure. Damn trash, I thought, and we could easily have taken that kit on our trip down the Current River, used its pot to boil crawdads or water for morning oatmeal. Just as easily saved a little money when times were tight for John and me, which I hadn't wanted to admit to my dad. We could also have saved some dollars if Dad had let me use those lumpy old flannel-lined sleeping bags for the kids. Into the trash. I saved the enamel cups with belt-hook handles for George, who swore they dated from one of Dad's 1930s climbing trips in the Alps.

I paused, recrossed my legs. Our parents' antiquated, state-of-the-art props for the outdoor life held for them the promise of yet another trip, the possibility of more mountains to explore, Dad's wish that Mom would relent and agree to sleep out under the stars one more time. Those musty sleeping bags with peeling, rubberized coatings enfolded memories I couldn't know—a night when my parents zipped together their bags into one warm cocoon, a night when August's shooting stars flashed across a black western sky and Dad elbowed Mom awake to witness the glory of the heavens—he surely would have used that biblical language. I needed a helmet to protect myself from memories of Dad as stingy and biblical.

The cedar blanket chest came next. As a child, I had loved to open and close the chest and inhale its fragrance. Blankets still lived here—one rough and drab from the Marine Corps; some yellowed ivory wool ones, monogrammed in navy wool with "1841" and "1843"; a loosely woven, rose-colored throw, for some reason "precious" to Mom; the Coleman coverlet from the homestead in Foristell, Missouri, or maybe even from Kentucky; and an afghan whose jewel-colored squares were crocheted together with black yarn. Nana Coleman had made one afghan for each of her two sons-in-law. As I lifted each blanket, moth crystals sprinkled onto the floorboards. Mom had added them ceremoniously every spring until recently. Oh, those blankets, what on earth would become of them? Would they ever be useful again? How could I get rid of their acrid pungency? Enough. I had no more decision making left in me that day.

The heat, the mix of cedar and mothball odors, and the weight of memories pushed me out of the attic, helmet in hand. I hauled one trash bag of Christmas tree lights and camping gear and leftover wrapping paper to the stairs. I hung my father's helmet on the hook by the attic door.

—⁓—

In November 2002, I wrote Missy in Colorado and George in Tuscany an update about Mom and her life with YumYum in Villa Manor. At our regular quarterly visit to her doctor in August, Mom had received permission to try to wean herself from her walker. She considered using it a sign of weakness. In hopes of independence, she undertook an intensive physical therapy program; Medicare would cover the cost as long as she made progress. Mom and the therapist worked on her balance and stability. She appeared to walk a little more steadily.

Nonetheless, when Mom completed the therapy, she had not made enough progress and still required a walker because 1) she had poor balance on uneven or unfamiliar surfaces; 2) she was easily distracted and lost her balance when she wasn't thinking about walking, a danger at social occasions outside Villa Manor; and 3) Mom's independence and safety were her primary, though sometimes contradictory, goals.

So, in spite of Mom's strong perception that using a walker equaled social stigma, her doctor required her to use it for outings. Within Villa Manor, she was permitted to use only a cane because the facility provided hallway railings, resting spots, and nursing staff. The Villa Manor therapist reported her assessment to Mom, her doctor, and me. Mom went back to receiving physical therapy twice a week to maintain the modicum of progress and confidence she had gained. Our cost was $30 per week for two 15- to 20-minute sessions once Medicare stopped covering therapy. Mom and I discussed the dangers of a fall and the responsibility that many felt for her safety. She was, nonetheless, embarrassed to have to use the walker.

For her 90 years, Mom was in good shape, I told Missy and George. But during that autumn of 2002, I was not in good shape. I felt guilty for not empathizing with Mom about her failure to wean herself from the walker. I did not take her complaints of boredom and lack of outings and good books seriously enough. To me, she sounded like the ennui-filled symbolist poet Mallarmé, who said, "I've read every book." Then I chastised myself for lacking compassion. She was, after all, my very old mother.

In early November, I took Mom on a round of doctors' visits—to the internist for the next quarterly check-up and to the urologist for urinary tract problems. In the urologist's exam room, I helped her undress, hoisted her onto the examining table and into stirrups to wait for the doctor. She was unsteady and frightened about going through the exam alone. I held her hand and found myself face-to-face with her privates as the doctor tested her urinary output. I ran her quarterly pacemaker check, using the phone that connected to a computer in her cardiologist's office. I held a magnet on Mom's pacemaker, embedded under the thin mottled skin of her upper left chest. Moistened electrodes attached to both wrists. When I replaced the phone receiver in its cradle, a computer took measurements, followed by a nurse on the line who said, "See you over the phone in three months." Mom liked the attention that the pacemaker test and the appointments provided. "They are dates on my dance card," she said.

When I wrote to Missy and George, my restraint reminded me of our stoic father. How could I have become like him? I had just jettisoned the props of his life from the attic and pitched most of them into the trash. How could I turn into my stiff-upper-lipped dad? In messages to my siblings that fall, I portrayed John's and my good times as counter-balancing what actually had been increasingly heavy loads of time and energy I'd spent on both mothers. On one weekend, John and I attended a multimedia art opening and an a cappella choir concert with friends, I took a walk with my friend Lillian, and John and I went out for dinner with another couple. I sent Missy high hopes for early snow in the San Juan Mountains in Colorado, where she was a ski instructor, and wished George a safe trip home from Italy.

By mid-November, Sandra dressed Silvia each morning and lifted her into a wheelchair, where she slumped forward to sleep for much of the day. Silvia became delusional and at times hostile. She hit at me two times in one afternoon. She moaned or screamed—nonverbal noises rather than words. A few days later, we learned that her body was fighting a urinary tract infection. After I listened to Sandra describe Silvia's symptoms, John and I requested she be examined by a doctor, who diagnosed the infection and prescribed antibiotics for it.

Just before Thanksgiving, we moved Silvia to a single room in the skilled nursing unit because she could no longer perform the activities of daily living (ADLs), such as dressing herself, handling personal hygiene, and transferring from bed to chair on her own. Occasionally, Silvia could feed herself, her last independent act. As we watched her decline into the fierce symptoms of late-stage Alzheimer's disease, I wondered where God was and what God meant by allowing such degradation of a once vigorous, alert person.

Looking after Silvia took John several hours almost every day—contacting her doctors, dealing with the bookkeeper, phoning various nursing home personnel, and listening to Sandra's report at the end of her shift five days a week. The relentless responsibilities for our mothers sapped us, siphoned away our energy and zest. When we "solved" one problem, we couldn't relax because we knew another crisis lurked. For John, each crisis elicited anger, usually shouted out to our kitchen walls; for me, every crisis brought rock-heavy sadness.

In the midst of six or seven hellish weeks with Silvia, YumYum bit Mom. The bite became infected. Mom and Yummy took over my life for several days, in spite of fundamental end-of-life issues we were facing with Silvia. I took Mom to the emergency room late on a November evening for intravenous antibiotics to control her cat-bite infection. I conferred with Villa Manor about whether the cat could remain in her room. I promised Villa Manor that YumYum would remain in "quarantine" in Mom's room. I loaded the cat into a carrier and drove her to the vet to be checked for disease, a county requirement after an animal bite. On the way home, Yummy squalled and pooped all over the carrier.

I could not sympathize with Mom's heartbreak at the thought of losing Yummy. She coupled tears with threats if Yummy couldn't stay with her. Caring for our old people was driving me crazy. I, an ordinary, grandmotherly, former French teacher, hauled a yowling Siamese cat to a vet miles away on a rainy November night because the blasted cat bit its 90-year-old owner! Nothing in my life, including our children's illnesses, accidents, and adolescent traumas, had prepared me for such a role. I was angry because I didn't even like Yummy, who was haughty and unpredictable. Yet, YumYum gave Mom a reason to live, as Silvia's plant care had shaped her days. Mom hurried back to her room after each meal to see Yummy. She ascribed human emotions and reactions to YumYum. Mom told me, "Yummy is the only one who understands me."

Although Mom was lucid and determined in her reaction to Yummy's bite and quarantine—much like Silvia's clarity when her son Albert died—she became fuzzier mentally. I visited some refurbished apartments on her floor and said,

"Mom, they've fixed up those little apartments on your floor." I settled in for a chat on a straight chair that Mom loved because she'd needle pointed its rose and green seat.

"What apartments?"

"Down the hall. They're cozy and freshly painted with little kitchens and living rooms. You might like more space."

"On my floor? Nicer than this room?"

"More spacious. It might feel homier for you and Yummy," I said.

"I don't want a kitchen or anything to do with kitchens and food. And I'm not interested in another home." Her mouth pursed in determination as she said this.

"I thought I'd give you an option."

"Do you remember our old house?"

"I do, Mom. You're lucky to have this picture of it on your wall."

"All that lovely lawn," she stroked Yummy, who was stretched on her lap. "And those trees: your father was so proud of those trees. He had the tree man come every spring."

"We had some great times there. Remember when Dad tried to barbecue and we played croquet on the lawn?"

"Our house was like an English manor, wasn't it? A grand place for the whole family." Her wispy voice floated in threads back to a long-ago era.

"So, you're not interested in a larger apartment, are you?"

"No, not at all."

Five weeks later, Mom showed me an article in the Villa Manor newsletter about the refurbished apartments on her floor.

"Don't they sound cunning?" she said.

"We talked about them last month," I answered.

"We did? About these very apartments?"

"Yes, Mom, we had a fine discussion."

"Well, I declare. I don't have any recollection of ever having heard about these apartments before."

We had entered a period when Mom operated in a zone where important issues, such as her health and her living space, became fuzzy-wuzzied. If I needed a clear report, I was no longer able to rely on her information. That slippery time thrust me back to Dad's literary question about the "reliable narrator." I'd said that if a storyteller or novelist, rather than being a reliable narrator, was unreliable, he or she would skew a tale, exaggerate some of its details, and shape the story to his or her self-interest. Mom had done just that with the issue of her walker. She claimed that the doctor and physical therapist had told her she no longer needed a walker. She was in a never-never land, a place where I had to be gentle but not trust her version of the story. I had blocked out any thoughts that Mom might be on the verge of dementia.

During several days in December, Silvia was in excruciating pain or in the last throes of Alzheimer's disease or both. John needed to find a way to manage her pain. He and I felt frustrated with the pain management of the skilled nursing providers. Silvia screamed, "Aiuto!" (the Italian word for "Help!") and shouted; she struck at people; she tore her hair. She was agitated and tried repeatedly to stand up as if to walk or to uncramp herself. When asked the source of her pain, she pointed to her pelvic area, not automatically to the hip broken in Rome years before. Even though Silvia had healed well, she'd developed arthritis and then a limp from that hip. At last, Silvia's doctor from the Washington University Memory and Aging Project, gave a "pain-free" directive to the nursing staff. This overrode any previous nursing home directives.

Several months before, after Silvia had fallen, the nursing home staff brought in a portable X-ray machine but found nothing damaged. Antibiotics had brought a recent urinary tract infection under control. Nobody could locate the cause of Silvia's pain. Yet, I assumed that she was in pain. She cried with despair as she shrank mentally, physically, and emotionally. Finding the source of the pain would involve tests, a hospital stay, or at least an outing to the doctor's office, but any change disoriented Silvia. We did not know what we would do with the results of tests. What was the source of the pain that tore through this once-elegant, lively woman? We opted against trying to find out and were thankful for new, stronger pain medication administered regularly.

As caregiver questions dominated John's and my breakfast and dinner conversations, I continued to write in the journal I'd begun years before. I recorded my anguish about how to treat the end of Silvia's life, now being played out in grotesque slow motion. Sadness swallowed me as I watched Silvia die and my mother fail.

In mid-December, John and I attended a routine Care Plan meeting about Silvia. Sandra no longer attended because she needed to stay with Silvia, and Luciana lived in Massachusetts. This meeting felt different because Claudia, the crisp director of nursing, had finally accepted but not yet warmed up to John and me. She concluded that Silvia was "miserable" (her exact word), that she suffered from "pain and dementia." One played off the other. Misery revealed pain, and pain caused misery. No one, she told us, could map the landscape Silvia was traversing nor when she would reach the end. I was heartbroken for John as he faced these bald facts. He was not a doctor nor a therapist nor a rabbi nor a sage. He wanted only one thing: to alleviate his mother's pain. He seldom laughed any more.

Led by Claudia, we and the staff changed course and agreed to certain noninvasive, in-house tests, and then, depending on results, treatment to follow. Everyone gave lip service to keeping Silvia pain-free, not waiting until she cried in anguish to give her medications. Again, we explained to the staff that the Italian word "aiuto" means "help." We learned that Alzheimer's patients may cry out without being in pain. I questioned how anyone could know because victims such as Silvia were truly nonverbal, even if they uttered words. Silvia's outbursts were, I thought, an existential scream for release. This meeting proved to be momentous because, for the first time, a group of professional staff talked to us about Silvia's death.

Claudia looked intently at John. "Your mother is not dying right now. Do you understand me?"

"Yes," John answered. "Explain how you will know when she is dying." He stopped his note taking.

"Our staff recognizes signs of dying. Refusal to eat. Near total unresponsiveness. An odor from the hands."

"When will it happen?" John jotted a few notes, returned Claudia's look simply.

"If you're lucky, she will die quickly from a stroke or a heart attack. But most Alzheimer's patients die from pneumonia or an infection, from their organs shutting down. That goes more slowly."

"Will I know when she is dying?"

The rest of us listened to the dialogue between Claudia and John.

"We will know, in all likelihood. We'll call you. We'll have another Care Plan meeting. You may decide to call in hospice to manage her care here."

"I want it to happen fast. I want her not to suffer," John said. "Please."

"We all want it to happen quickly now," Claudia responded.

When we left, John stroked his mother's arm as she slumped in her wheelchair. He bent down in hopes she would smile at him or show a bit of recognition in her eyes. I marveled at John's unflinching faithfulness to his mother. This remarkable son, with all his fierce talk in our kitchen, touched the sagging skin of his beloved mamma's forearm as her flat hazel eyes fixed a point in some far distance.

A week after our Care Plan meeting, John had his second auto accident within four months. It was his fault. He called the accident "a lapse in judgment." There were no injuries in his collision with a Mack truck loaded with dirt. Yet, later a doctor would consider John's two accidents as evidence of some kind of seizure disorder.

John needed a protective helmet. So did I.

11

Escape to Safety
2003

During the winter of 2003, Mom said she felt as dreary as the season. Pain shot through her feet and heels at night, she went on too few outings, and she found all the Villa Manor meals tasteless and monotonous. During one of my visits, I mentioned that it would be fun to look forward to her 75th high school reunion, coming in the spring.

"I'm not sure I'll be here any longer," she said morosely.

"What are you thinking of, Mom?" I sensed us moving into a conversation about her death. I steadied myself. This terrain, which we'd visited occasionally in chats about her funeral and burial wishes, made me uneasy. That my mom would actually die remained foreign and scary to me, even surreal. Her daily, late afternoon phone calls were full of wry commentary on the nonagenarian life, laments about Villa Manor, and her need for me now, as I had once depended on her—Mom's calls and needs spun the fabric of my life those days. I felt as close to her as I could ever remember.

"I feel as if something will happen fast, and I won't be here," said my mother.

Then I said, almost involuntarily: "It wouldn't be so bad if it just happened fast."

She agreed. We both knew the "it" was her death, but that winter day neither of us would name it. As I drove home, my emotions were scrambled: sadness for myself without her in the future; hope that she would not suffer or linger like Silvia; desire that she indeed hurry up and die soon, so that so much of my life wouldn't be taken up by her care. Guilt, self-pity, affection, and a sense of duty roiled around inside me.

I felt as dreary and isolated as she did.

George, Missy, and the bank trust officer decided that we should terminate our contract with Donna, Mom's sleek, businesslike social worker. We never learned why Mom decided she no longer needed Donna's counseling or therapy. A few days before, Mom had begun to complain about Donna to the family. Donna phoned me, as she always did after one of their outings, to report that Dorothy had been hostile and short with her, a behavior change Donna found strange. She could not recall saying anything that might have offended or upset Dorothy. My siblings disapproved of Donna's charges for "counseling" and "therapeutic" excursions that lasted several hours and frequently included lunch. I, however, relied on Donna as a sounding board for my concerns about Mom's well-being. Donna also charged her phone sessions with me to our family account. Though I valued Donna's steady guidance, I was outnumbered and designated by the family to let her go. I wrote a script, practiced it with John, and settled at my desk on a winter Monday morning, determined to go through with the dreaded task. The phone rang; it was Donna.

"Susan, I've been thinking," she began, "that your mother can't accept my help any more. She is very rude to me. I have no idea why she's turned against me." Donna used almost the same words I had written in my script.

"I've been hearing that, too," I said.

"If she shuts down, I'm no longer able to help her."

"The family thinks the same thing."

"You know, Susan, how fond I am of your mother, how many important times we've shared. I've counseled her through your father's death, her grief, her pacemaker, and her move."

"Donna, I'm so grateful for your help to Mom and to me—you've kept me steady, too."

"We have come to the end of this relationship." Donna did not want to linger; her tone was businesslike. "I'll send you a final invoice at the end of the month. Wish your mother well for me."

"Calling you was first on my list this morning. You beat me to it. The family agrees that we're at the end of this phase. Thank you, thank you, Donna."

"I read the obituaries every day. But give me a call, please, when your mother goes."

So ended our relationship with Donna.

"Goodbye," I said. I felt terrible in every way. I didn't like being backed into doing something I didn't agree with. I hated firing helpers. I wished I'd communicated more clearly to Missy and George how valuable Donna's support had been to me. But I had to move on, to handle crises with as much good humor and wisdom as I could muster. I would turn to John and friends and walks with our dog, Rufus, for my comfort and support.

Some light moments lifted my winter doldrums. The mobile and cognitively able residents at Villa Manor ate in an airy dining room with bay windows and French doors that opened onto a patio. Tables were set for from one to four people, spaced to allow for walkers and wheelchairs. When Mom moved to Villa Manor in March 2002, she had told the social director who assigned tables that she wanted to eat alone. I conferred with the director about Mom's self-decreed isolation and about her scorn for other residents, whom she called "old cripples" or "inmates." The social director felt that she should accede to Mom's request. She would, instead, try to engage Mom in other activities, such as the Current Affairs Club.

In February 2003, however, life in the dining room promised a change for my mom. Sally, who had grown up near Mom in St. Louis's Central West End, decided to move from Villa Manor to Florida for the climate and proximity to one of her children. In pink and yellow resort clothes, Sally sat with her apartment door open, at work on her computer. In the dining room, Sally held forth at a table Mom said had lots of "jollification" and included one man. Men, especially sentient men, were a rarity at Villa Manor, as they were at Silvia's, Paul's, and Dad's nursing homes. The man, Judge Lodge, conferred impressive social cachet on Sally's table. When the group scouted for Sally's replacement, Sally mentioned to Mom that she was a candidate for the table. Judge Lodge himself thought Mom might fit in. One day the judge spoke with Mom to ascertain that she was indeed George's widow and to proffer his own credentials as a retired federal judge.

That same February on a Wednesday afternoon, Mom decided that I could help her order a spring suit from a catalog. The promise of the new dining room table assignment pushed her to spruce herself up and break the grip of February melancholy, the month of Dad's birthday and death, a month flooded with memories of celebrations and trips to Arizona to escape the cold, plans for tree trimming and springtime planting at their house on Ballas Road.

The alterations on the suit were daunting. Its pants were cut to ride low over a smooth, 30-year-old stomach, not to fit a 90-year-old whose inseam was distorted by adult diapers. Mom refused to give up and said tartly that she would wear different underpinnings, "as long as I am not going to be out long." Female vanity drove her to flexibility. Elke, our Bosnian seamstress with a broad smiling face, squeezed around the walker in the fitting room, gently coached Mom to stand up as straight as possible to be measured, and suggested with a twinkle that Mom might like to try a funky, crinkly top.

Elke remade the pants so that they fit. But the alterations nearly doubled their cost. When we picked the suit up, Mom took out a check, wrote the number digits, raised her head, looked directly at me, and said, "I can't spell the numbers for the next line." Without a word, I filled out the rest of the check.

Stunned and shaken by my mom's new failing, I left her walker on the curb by Elke's shop. I worried that my own check-writing capacity might slip away and that my faculties would all slip, as my parents' had. I was overwhelmed by the vulnerabilities evident in Mom's decline, leavened with her springtime vanity and gutsiness. I felt threatened by a future just like her old age.

After settling Mom back into her room without her walker, I walked down the Villa Manor hall after that Wednesday fitting. Two ladies, each with neatly curled gray hair, sat on a window seat by the nurses' station.

The first lady said, "You know, I just get so confused these days. It worries me."

Lady Two nodded with empathy. "I understand exactly."

"Well, for example, I don't even know what day it is today."

Lady Two replied with quiet assurance: "I can help on that. It is

Friday."

The first lady sighed, "Oh, I'm so relieved to know."

I trudged to my car, wondering what world I lived in: a suit rebuilt to honor the spring and Mom's renewed desire to be attractive; a walker I forgot because I was sad and startled that Mom couldn't write simple words. I drove back to Elke's, picked up the walker, and delivered it to Villa Manor so Mom would have it to go to the dining room for dinner. Checking a wall calendar, I reassured myself that it was, indeed, Wednesday.

Just before Mom's March 4th birthday, I took her for a regular checkup with her internist. She showed no changes other than a fifteen-pound weight loss in the last year, which the doctor attributed to "social reasons." Mom continued to miss my father's company and to grieve his death. On her ninetieth birthday, she decided to give up driving—my siblings and I had been on the cusp of taking away her driving privileges—and the independence it offered. Her move from a large, gracious house to a small apartment marked a further narrowing of her life. She no longer had a kitchen, where she could pick up a piece of fudge or a handful of crackers each time she passed through.

While we waited an hour for the doctor, Mom told me stories about her father, my Granddaddy Coleman. Granddaddy was always referred to around St. Louis as the Judge because he was a judge. Even though I called him Granddaddy, I was as much in awe of him as others appeared to be. When he asked to see my fingernails to make sure I didn't bite them, I was terrified. I didn't bite them, but I feared they would appear too short. I loved how commanding Granddaddy was as he drove me to the Botanical Garden in his large, gray sedan with slippery leather seats. He asked me to spell "chrysanthemum." I couldn't and still can't. While I hated that moment, I loved how bluff and big Granddaddy was, especially his huge, shiny bald head. My brother George was now as tall as but slimmer than Granddaddy, with the same handsome, bare head.

In the doctor's office, Mom lay on the examining table with a blue smock over her chest, a sheet on her legs, and bare feet sticking out. In a flash, I glimpsed her as if she were lying there dead. I watched her lie perfectly still as family anecdotes floated out like bubbles, then drifted away, shrinking or popping as they disappeared. Miniature, evanescent legacies burst over her: there was Uncle Hal, Granddaddy Coleman's youngest brother, who, like Granddaddy, left the family farm near the rural town of Foristell, Missouri, to seek his fortune in St. Louis.

"A sweet guy, but no-account. Uncle Hal, he didn't get in trouble with the bottle or with women; he just couldn't hold a job," Mom said. She gazed straight up at the acoustic tiles as if to conjure kin from the bumps and crevasses of the ceiling.

"By the way," Mom asked me, "do you know what happened to the picture of me on the steps of our house with Uncle Trout? Old Uncle Trout used to appear for Sunday dinner. It was the Great Depression. All the country kinfolk landed at our house. In the snapshot, I was about 16 and wearing an ermine stole. I was really set up by that stole."

Granddaddy Coleman came from a sprawling family with names like Walter Dan and Trout. He had three sisters, Jessie, Mary, and Anna. He named his own first daughter Jessie Mary Anna. That was my late aunt— my favorite Aunt Mamie, who lived in Boston and spent summers on Cape Cod. Her son, Lanny, came to Mom's ninetieth birthday party. Nana Coleman, the judge's wife, got naming rights for their second daughter, my mother, Dorothy Jean.

Mom chuckled down deep in her chest from the doctor's table: "Aunt Jessie—you never knew my aunt. She was the one who sent us kids into gales of laughter when she came to visit. At night she hung her wig on the bedstead. We all wanted to sneak in and touch it. She was an evangelist, went around preaching the gospel." Jessie had married a Monser, Mom explained. "The Monsers went out to Kansas City, but Jessie's husband died young. He was no good. They didn't have any children."

Mom's reminiscing rolled on as she lay on the examining table; she laced her tales with folksy Missouri expressions that she used only when she was in her Coleman frame of mind: "no-account, no good, trouble with the bottle." How far this seemed from the austere, elegant drawing rooms full of unspoken intrigue and wartime sorrow in John's family's palazzi on the Grand Canal in Venice.

When she paused, I told Mom I'd read a Civil War novel by Paulette Jiles called *Enemy Women*. The primary story line is fictional, but the outline is based on real events and people in the Ozarks, St. Louis, and points in between. Among the bands of outlaws hidden in the Ozarks was a Coleman group. I asked Mom if these renegades were related to our family's Colemans.

"You're asking me whether the Colemans were Southern sympathizers. Now, I don't think so. They were feisty sorts and already in Missouri by the time of the Civil War, farming out in Foristell. Remember that coverlet from Foristell—that blue and white one with a different pattern on each side? Hard to make, you know. Well, that came from Kentucky with them, just like that old walnut spool dresser you have. They settled down. The Colemans weren't in the Ozarks." Her eyes closed so that her forebears could visit, I imagined. She clucked with pride. "Or at least, I don't think they were bandits. But I can't be sure."

As for me, I wanted my Coleman ancestors to have been untamed, independent Ozark outlaws!

Mom dozed, her feet straight up. Those big, bony Coleman feet— Kentucky, Ozark, and Foristell, Missouri, feet—I shared those. Good feet for balance on Ozark ridge paths and on rocky fords across mountain rivers, like the Jack's Fork and the Huzzah. Fine feet for rebels or even for city firebrands, as my mom had proved herself to be over and over in women's reproductive rights battles.

Three days later, Mom turned 91. We gave a dinner party at our house for her with John and me, George and Gabriele, and Betty T. The table with our best china and crystal, a lamb roasted pink on the inside and crisp on the outside, and candles lighting salmon-colored roses—my mother's favorite flowers—all made for a festive setting. Betty brought the senior yearbook from the girls' school she and Mom had attended. After dinner, as we sat by the fire, Betty read the kudos under Mom's flapper-style photo:

"Dorothy Coleman, editor of the newspaper, winner of the junior book prize, captain of the field hockey team, student government representative."

"Wow, were you ever versatile!"

"Amazing, Mom." I rarely thought of my mother as a teenager. Yet, I had a dozen formal studio portraits of Mom after high school, lined up in our basement, where, from time to time, Missy and I tried to assign dates to them. Engagement or college senior picture or newspaper photo to accompany her occasional byline: a coy tilt of the head; Marcel waves; soft, round cheeks; intense eyes; dark, naturally arced eyebrows. I noticed my mother's eyebrows because they contrasted with mine that were so fair they were invisible. Our daughter Ellen mailed me an eyebrow enhancer wand when I lamented my case. Mom still had bushy, expressive eyebrows. The clothes in her photo portraits were scrumptious. Even in black and white, the shimmer of satin, a mink-collared wrap, and folds of artfully draped necklines spoke drama and luxury.

Betty went on: "Now here are all Dorothy's theater credits. Look at these shots of her playing Medea." Betty held up the yearbook for us to admire.

"Here it says," Betty continued, "Dorothy Coleman, vice-president, class of 1928."

We oohed and aahed at Mom's achievements. Mom dropped her eyes theatrically.

Betty cleared her throat: "And I, Betty, was president of the class of 1928."

I laughed as Mom's oldest friend tweaked her, reminding me of the lifelong devotion and competition between the two. The rivalry dated back to when they began grade five together in the early 1920s. The evening ended with Mom, Betty, and me singing camp songs from Northway Lodge, a Canadian wilderness camp attended by three generations of girls—Mom, Aunt Mamie, and Betty; Missy and me; and our daughter Carol.

"We're the Namagoochees who camped on the Boncheres; oh, we're the Namagoochees of 1-9-2-4. Head Lake to Boundary. . . ." and on through a list of lakes, canoe portages, and streams that Betty and Mom sang out in raspy cheer. I joined in as the words came back to me. In my 1950s-era camp, we adapted the close harmony of the sh-boom, sh-boom type for songs to memorialize our canoe trip adventures. George, in his melodious tenor voice, hummed along, as his partner Gabriele and John must have wondered at this loyalty to an adolescent wilderness camp experience, seventy-five years ago for Mom and Betty, forty-five years ago for me.

The fire crackled. Mom carried the bouquet of roses home with her.

Betsy from New York and various cousins remembered Mom's birthday with calls and cards. For her dinner party at our house, she had worn a new black crepe dress with a jacket that she pronounced her "laying-out" dress. She said she wanted to practice wearing it and getting the accessories right.

—∿—

The day after Mom's 91st birthday, we had a quarterly Care Plan meeting at Silvia's nursing home. We had sensed hints of coming trouble from several phone calls: Silvia had banged on the dining room table, pinched and scratched staff members, held and then kissed hands. She shouted and demanded attention, as if to say, 'Please, please, oh please, help me somehow.' So John and I rehearsed the meeting on our morning walk. Obsessed, we stamped along our neighborhood sidewalks, parallel figures, eyes on the ground, role-playing, as we spoke out to the brilliant forsythia, the budded dogwood trees, the daffodils bold yellow on their stalks. We explored the possibilities, with the worst scenario that the director would ask us to move Silvia from the facility, just as Paul had been forced to move from his first placement because of violent behavior.

Our Care Plan meeting began with politeness and restraint that skirted Silvia's behavioral problems. I sat patiently through the calorie intake, weight report, and activity participation barometer.

"Yes, Sandra wheels Silvia into the song programs," said the activity director. "Sometimes Silvia sleeps. Recently, she has been yelling, so we've asked Sandra to take her back to her room."

"We should tell you that some residents' families complain about how loud your mother's screams are. The families hear the screams as they come in the door," Claudia, the head nurse, said.

No report from physical therapy, still financed by our family, because Silvia dozed in her wheelchair during each session.

I read the chief of nursing's watch upside down: 9:50 a.m. We had until ten o'clock.

"Excuse me," I ventured. John and I had planned this. We presumed my words and my tone might be more neutral because Silvia was my mother-in-law. Yet, I knew what the staff did not: Silvia had touched my life deeply with her survival techniques, her grit, her inventiveness, her nurture. She awoke none of the ambiguities that my mother's dramatic, vigorous, and imperious persona evoked in me.

"You know, John and I have been wondering," I spoke slowly, "about whether you all have adequate facilities to take care of Silvia in her present state. We were just wondering."

Claudia cleared her throat. "Yes, well. That's a question we have asked ourselves."

John looked up from his notes.

9:53 a.m.

I wondered why we had spent so much time covering all that weight, dietary, and programmatic material.

I couldn't let myself begin to criticize. Eye on the ball . . . Silvia's care . . . Silvia's screams . . . Silvia's pain . . . and her comfort. John and I couldn't begin to hunt for a new nursing home. Keep writing, John. Don't scowl. Let them talk, talk themselves into their own competence: "Oh yes, of course we can deal with her; we've seen worse. After all, it is our job to care for people, for people with all sorts of diseases."

Their voices invaded me.

"But, perhaps, come to think of it, now that we put the pieces together, you know, all along we have been thinking Silvia might do better in a different room on a corridor with the highest level of specialized care. Why yes, of course, we have a room for her. Just what we had in mind, just what we were coming to, so kind of you, insightful even, to bring this to our attention. Thank you."

9:57 a.m.

Silvia would have to move immediately to a still higher level of care, where there were fewer social expectations, for example, at meals, and activities were geared not to cognitive skills but to the five senses. The activity director explained them as smelling and touching. Even then, I didn't understand why Silvia needed to develop her senses. I thought these activities sounded like torture for an immobile, nonverbal old lady who suffered from terminal Alzheimer's disease.

In our last few minutes, the conversation veered, as it had in December, to Silvia's dying. I never dreamed that I would participate in conversations about a family member's death, that this would be the focal point of my late middle life, that the man I married for love and fun and adventure—my husband of thirty-eight years—would articulate a desire for his adored mother's death. To my shock, I, too, wished that Silvia would die soon. But with these professional caregivers around, I was engulfed by shame. I discussed my reactions with John—hope for death followed by guilt. John had journeyed through that stage. He was calm in the confidence that over the last few years he had given all he could and had left no caregiving stone unturned. I still agonized.

That week in March epitomized my life in the middle of the very old mothers as they lived and declined. I yo-yoed between sharing the pleasure Mom drew from her new suit and her birthday festivities and worry over care for Silvia. Though Mom wasn't chosen for the table with the judge, her winter gloom lifted, thanks to longer days, a flowering Bradford pear tree outside her window, and her new outfit. In contrast, Silvia's spirit had either disappeared or become locked within her because of Alzheimer's disease.

Before I'd retired from teaching, I viewed myself as about to begin my "real adulthood," a life of my own choices with the blessings of wisdom, experience, and good health. I joshed with friends about what I was going to be when I grew up. I didn't realize that my maturing had already

started. I had, it seemed, chosen caregiving, or rather, it had chosen me
for this period of life that author Abigail Trafford calls *My Time*. Trafford postulates a two- or three-decade bubble for people my age, an era
of expansion, "generativity," contribution, and fulfillment. Yet, she does
not take into account the situations or duties that choose us.

When Paul was diagnosed with Alzheimer's disease, the choosing
began. Even before his diagnosis, I had heard Sharon, who became my
in-laws' case manager, speak at my church about dealing with old parents.
Until Sharon's talk, our four parents' aging hadn't overtly affected me.
Sharon enumerated early signs of Alzheimer's disease: anger, forgetful-
ness, poor judgment, suspicion. True, Paul had begun to hide money and
valuables, lose keys, and wander. I found myself taking notes intently, as I
stitched together Paul's behaviors into an amateur diagnosis of what was
still a mysterious, yet feared disease. I latched onto this newfound knowledge and recognition about Paul. Caregiving for our parents selected
me—an accident of geography, of showing up by chance. At that Sunday
church meeting, without realizing what I was doing, I made a commit-
ment to John's and my parents as they set out on the final stages of life.

I didn't know whether John had experienced an epiphany or commit-
ment to our caregiving role. He usually invoked duty and responsibility, as
if caregiving followed logically. By nature, he was not prone to stand back
and analyze. He didn't discuss whether caring for our aged parents had
shaped our personalities and our life together. Instead, he asserted that
caring for our parents would not keep us from our own lives. Neither of
us wanted to face how much caregiving had molded us, had become our
life. Yet, as if we intuited the impact of our parents' old age, I continued
to chronicle daily events, our parents' evolving symptoms, and John's
and my reactions and emotions. Perhaps I hoped that in the writing, I
would create a talisman against the same ravages in our old age, for John

and I vowed that we would not afflict our children with such caregiving responsibilities.

At the watershed moment of my mother's birthday and a change in Silvia's Care Plan, I recognized that I was more thoughtful, subdued, and sad than in the past. I wondered if this season was 'rock bottom,' a depth of helplessness to which I'd never fallen before. Once in awhile, when called on another "mercy mission," I found myself crying as I drove to Villa Manor or Silvia's nursing home. I hated my self-pity. Even though I had chosen a caregiving role for our four parents, I didn't realize that the process might launch me on the path to old age myself. Along the way, I had missed the grace period—the period of grace when John and I would have been at full capacity mentally, physically, and emotionally and comfortable in our resources and our children and their futures. John missed it even more than I. His father's death had been rugged and strung out. His mother was gravely ill with Alzheimer's disease. His younger brother Albert's death was a blow to his heart. John's own undefined illness troubled him deeply. Yet, in spite of every new complexity and unexplained symptom, he pushed on with fierce family loyalty. I loved John all the more for his steady devotion to his parents and his love and support for me.

I went to see Daniel, my pastor, the only representative of God I knew to consult. I hoped he would know whether the pieces of this fragmented, doleful period of my life composed a pattern, a story if viewed differently. Daniel would discern, perhaps, what God had in store for me. True, I found that if I sat in silence, tuned out the world, listened inwardly—prayed, some might call it—I could prepare for the day ahead. But in my heart, during the days of Alzheimer's dying, I wondered where God was, why deaths piled one on top of the other, why John fell, afflicted by his maladies, why I found myself in the midst of woes. I had to ask someone.

Best it be Pastor Daniel, about 40 years old, crew-cut hair, wild wide ties, aficionado of the sixties and Martin Luther King, Jr.

I thought I knew in advance how our conversation would unfurl. I could plot the steps on a chart. The instructions to a counselor, therapist, social worker, professor, or pastor were to listen actively, affirm, recognize, acknowledge, validate, lean in, nod, listen again, press the tips of the fingers together, no need to speak. Make known the seriousness of the petitioner's dilemma. I doubted that Daniel or any living being could explain God's role. God didn't have time for the neuritic plaques and neurofibrillary tangles of Alzheimer's disease.

Goddamn you, God, you ought to have time to be here for me! What kind of God floats around up there in Tiepolo baby-blue clouds with angels in attendance on a ceiling? That's no God, who won't even give me a little break, maybe a week off in Mexico. I would bargain for three days with a promise to get back in the saddle, go full steam ahead, any expression you choose, if I could have a few days off, with no worry about John having another seizure when he goes blank, stumbles, babbles, and falls asleep; when I don't have to drive him anywhere; when the phone doesn't ring, 'Hello, this is the charge nurse the charge nurse the charge nurse'; when I don't have to stop by just for a moment: oh please hold my hand, bring me some chocolate and, yes, some kitty litter, do you mind just stopping by? Why doesn't God liberate me for time with my kids and grandkids, whisk me away for hugs and stories from Pooh and diaper genies and soy formula in strange cities where no one knows me and I can bring pure, singleminded, attentive love to these young families?

"So I came today, Daniel, to see what all this caregiving means? And John's illness? And my role? Basically, why me?"

"I hear you." We sat face to face, our knees nearly touching in his book-filled office.

"What does God mean by it? How can John and I ever choose hospice care for Silvia? I don't believe we can decide on our own that it's the end of Silvia's life. I don't believe in it."

"Tell me about her."

"She's not Silvia any more. Even God wouldn't recognize her. I counted—she stood up and down thirty times in her wheelchair when I visited her yesterday. Then tried to pinch me. Then slumped over and fell fast asleep."

Daniel ran his hand over his crew cut. "You know that the hospice people do their own analysis?"

"That's not the point. Who gives me or anyone else the right even to consider letting Silvia die?"

We sat quietly for a moment. I hoped Daniel was interceding for me with God.

"Susan, God says to Moses before he can approach the burning bush, 'Take off your sandals because you are standing on holy ground' [Exodus 3:5]. You and John are walking on holy ground as you make this journey of dying with your parents. Holy ground, life and death. I hope you know that." He was quiet for a moment. "Would you like us to pray together?"

—⁂—

Hell, "sandals off for holy ground?" What's that about? Am I meant to wear that verse like a charm? Shall I murmur "holy ground" as a mantra to remind myself when Sandra calls about Silvia pinching a nurse's aide; when my mother complains about the paltry food and devil-may-care table service; when a doctor asks me to decide, to choose, to just say 'yes' or 'no' to lipivascaramotobolic at 50 milligrams more a day it will have a soothing or diuretic or waking or constipating or soporific effect. The charm of holy ground will carry me forward—is that how it will work if I take off my sandals, Pastor Daniel? Plead for me loudly in your prayer, Daniel. I need "it," whatever it is. I can barely walk through each day, much less navigate holy ground.

And yet, I remembered that for a sweet moment, I had known holiness as I sat alone next to Paul's body at 3 a.m. in the sterile hospital room, as I muttered last words to his turbulent, vivacious spirit. It had been sacred when I told my father, ever so gently, that I couldn't help him go home any faster to his mother and father and sister. Yet, I did hold his hand until death rattled through his thin frame and stilled him—that was holy. Now the mothers. I was exhausted.

—⁂—

In spite of the new gray worsted suit specially tailored for her, my mother could no longer keep up the grooming standards she set for herself. Sometimes she was too stiff to bend over and work stockings up her legs. Zippers, buttons, and the clasps on jewelry demanded too much dexterity from her knotted, arthritic fingers. I had helped with alterations, and now I was shopping with her for clothes and makeup. I was struck on an outing by our newfound intimacy, for we had seldom shared shopping before. The narrator in Proust's *The Captive* has a moment when, thanks to observing a minute detail, he, too, grasps the intimacy of having lured his mistress, Albertine, into living with him. I recognized my entwinement with my mother at a cosmetics counter in a department store. Mom held out her green plastic lipstick case:

"I'd like another just like this. It's called 'Ginger Flower.'"

As in the moments when, at age 9 or 10, I tested her theater makeup, I had a flash of insight into Mom's enduring sense of herself as womanly, attractive, dramatic. By knowing the name of the color she wore on her lips, I knew her, was entwined in a profound way, like Proust's narrator with Albertine. In *The Captive*, the narrator says, "A little later Albertine took to wearing slippers, some of gold kid, others of chinchilla, the sight of which gave me great pleasure because they were all of them signs . . . that she was living under my roof." A mistress's slippers served as an emblem of their cohabitation. My mother's lipstick, "Ginger Flower," whose name bore the exotic perfume of India, the poignant promise of blossom, of transformation, reassured me that at last, in my sixties, I shared one totem of her charm.

—⁓—

At the end of April, John burst into the kitchen: "I pulled the plug on my mother today."

I jumped up and hugged him; then began to tremble inside myself. I hated that language. I hated the decision about someone else's life. My husband suddenly seemed foreign to me.

John had engaged a hospice service to take over Silvia's nursing care, with Sandra's continued assistance as private caregiver. We understood that hospice's policy was to cease curative measures and to use only palliative care to keep Silvia comfortable and free of pain. The Hospice Foundation of America's website states, "Hospice election is a choice that means accepting death and giving up aggressive treatment." Hospice directions would now supersede those of the nursing home staff, though Silvia remained there. As Silvia's dying progressed, the hospice staff offered services to John and me and to Sandra, such as opportunities to meet with a social worker, attend grieving groups, and schedule consultations with their charge nurses. John and I frequently consulted with the hospice nurses and administrators caring for Silvia. We did not, however, avail ourselves of their counseling or spiritual services because we felt surrounded by strong friends, family, and helpmates.

My pastor's words rang in my ears: oh yes this is sacred ground take off your sandals humble yourself fall face down in hope that providence or grace will lift you up in hope in hope. But I could not have felt any lower than I felt in the spring of 2003.

Silvia—my God, that last month, those last two years of her life, our life, all of our lives were miserable. Before John selected hospice services, a nursing home psychiatrist and the nursing staff had tried a variety of medication cocktails to control Silvia's behavior, alleviate her pain, and keep her conscious some of the time. Because the nursing home was committed to cures, they treated bowel and bladder infections aggressively until hospice took over. Silvia descended deeper and deeper into a zone where neither John nor I could rouse her to lift her head. Once in a rare while, she opened her eyes; she often shouted, "Aiuto." Sandra said that she widened her mouth for food without lifting her head or opening her eyes, like the automatic reflex of a baby bird.

Luciana came to visit Silvia in April, many months after her previous visit, when she had felt so hurt by Silvia's failure to recognize her that she could not bring herself to face her mother. Since that earlier visit, Luciana had offered John a listening ear; she phoned often to learn how Silvia was, offering John understanding, gratitude for looking after their mother, and no criticism of his decisions.

By April 2003, I resented the circumstances that had thrust John and me into nearly ten years of caregiving for his parents. As I think about that spring, I have to admit to being ashamed of myself for those feelings.

Silvia seemed lost to us already. Spring had been her season to bloom. In spring, the pink dogwood tree Silvia had saved by drastic pruning announced its survival with new blossoms. Walking our dog in years past, I would find Silvia kneeling in the garden, gloved hands in the soil she had enriched over the years. In early summer, Silvia moved the big potted plants outside, set out her basil seedlings, and readied the pool for lazy afternoons of chat about children and world affairs. Silvia would never have wanted to endure springtime in a nursing home. Now, taking care of her meant letting her go, allowing her to die.

John's anxieties about his mother and his own health intensified that spring's problems. He had new medications: one for partial seizure epilepsy, his diagnosis after 18 months of tests and uncertainty, and one to guard against mood swings—particularly depression or sleeplessness— which can precipitate seizures. Merciful God, I thought, John needs some relief. It was hard for me to remember the John of enthusiasm and picnics with special Italian food, of corny jokes and brisk walks together.

John's diagnosis included a six-week moratorium on driving, until the doctor felt confident that his medications would prevent further seizures. Daily, I became part of his doctor's orders—no driving until May 28, on the condition that John was seizure-free until then. So I drove. John hated my driving—the way I drove, the routes I chose, the car's speed, the temperature setting. I understood that what he really hated was his loss of independence. He shouted at me, "If you don't go my way, well then, I'm just going to take the car and. . . ." He was frightened: afraid of his mother's death, concerned for his own health, and, like me, worried that his future held Alzheimer's disease. Again, as when I alerted my siblings to the danger of our parents' falls, I had to play the role of the bad cop, only this time for my husband.

—∿—

After a family brunch in mid-May, Mom said, as I drove her home, "I do get mixed up with all the generations and families."

"Well, Mom," I temporized.

"Now, remind me, this party you had was for . . . for?"

"For Anna, Mom, Missy's daughter. For her college graduation."

"Anna. Oh, yes."

Mom had used her "summoning voice," the one she used when she called up her ancestors. How could she let her dear St. Louis grandchild, Anna, slip away? Anna, with her whimsical spirit, had taken a Jane Austen DVD and some homemade supper to entertain her grandmother on a Sunday evening. Anna often brought Mom relief from charge nurses and aides, inattentive servers and pill monitors; Anna also brought Mom relief from me, ever vigilant about her well-being and seldom amusing. I counted on Anna, who had stayed in St. Louis to attend college when Missy and Walt moved to Colorado. Mom loved her youngest grand-daughter, the grandchild who had given hours of happy distraction to her grandmother.

"Missy, now who is Missy?"

"Missy is my sister and your younger daughter. She's Anna's mother. That's why Missy came to town. For Anna's graduation." There I went, straightening my mom out—reaching into my sadness in hopes that I could align her with the facts and slow down her confusion.

Mom went on, "Oh yes. Well, was she at your house today?"

"Yes, Mom, Missy was there the whole time."

"I don't remember seeing her. What was she wearing?"

"A long navy dress with a little print on it. Remember, she gave a toast to Anna at the table."

Mom answered, "Oh yes, she was there to my left." She peered ahead at the road, as if a picture of the family around the table would rise up before her.

"Right, Mom." I answered with a rock of sorrow in the pit of my stomach.

During that visit, Missy saw Mom as a standard 91-year-old. But I couldn't dismiss our mother as standard. I wanted to talk with my sister about buying Mom's lipstick and fitting her spring suit. I needed to wonder aloud with Missy about whether we sisters would have skin as dry and tissue-thin as Mom's or would be just as stubborn and tenacious about the graceful things in life, such as manicured nails and new seasonal outfits. I could have tried to explain how Mom resonated with me—how I heard angst in her voice or noticed unusual odors or spots on her clothes, how my antennae were out for signs of change. I longed for a back and forth, detailed conversation about mother-daughter relationships with Missy. "Relationship talk" wasn't John's realm, especially not in this season of his own anguish. Yet, I was lucky that Missy and George accepted my role in our mother's care, just as Luciana had never second-guessed John's decision making about their parents. In our joint efforts, we tried not to lose sight of maintaining close relations during the final years of our parents' lives and thereafter.

—⁓—

Six weeks after John gave Silvia over to hospice care, she hung on peacefully. The hospice staff brought practicality and compassion to her care, which showed on her smooth face. Hospice prescribed peace: simplicity with no stimulation, no pretense about connection with her surroundings, and no medications except for morphine to keep her comfortable. The hospice nurses vetoed nursing home attempts at dining room meals or social activities. Instead, Silvia lay clean and virtually naked in her bed. Her reactions to the outside world vanished. No life lines or recipe codes attached her to the world she had inhabited. John reflected her calm in this final stage of his mother's life. He and I felt relieved not to have to confront the nursing home staff about jovial care, relieved that Silvia appeared comfortable in her darkened room with photos of Paul and her children, etchings of Venice, and furniture from Italy around her.

Silvia lay in bed, shifted slightly by a nurse onto one side or the other every few hours. She moaned softly, "Aiuto," then slipped back into herself. She opened her mouth for Sandra to feed her a spoonful of pureed peaches, a bit of yogurt, some meat blended with potatoes, a swallow of cranberry juice. Usually, the food lay inert on her lips and tongue, then drooled down her chin. Her collarbones stuck out from the hospital gown, her only garment. In mid-June, she began to clench her hands, which sweated a little, into balls. A sour odor of death came from her hands—hands that once knitted a sweater for a grandchild in a few weeks and rolled out dough for pasta frolla shortbread cookies and pinched back basil so that it grew on and on into the fall for a winter's supply of pesto; strong hands that wrote coded recipes, stirred risotto, dipped film into chemicals, raised her children.

Our children said goodbye. They whispered into Silvia's ear and hoped for a reaction, such as a blink or a nod. One by one, they came from her room in tears, then flew to their far-flung homes. Luciana had said goodbye on her April visit. John's sister-in-law Lynn and her children planned to pay tribute at whatever gathering we held after Silvia's death. John and I said goodbye every evening.

Silvia herself no longer existed. The last kiss I gave Silvia on her waxen forehead—not a blink of an eye, not a movement, almost no warmth to that forehead—was like kissing a corpse. One day her waxy skin was splotched, another day yellowish, but it looked dead. Curiously, her wrinkles softened away. When she was resting with her mouth closed, her chest moving evenly up-down-up-down, she looked as if she had washed up on another shore where she was welcomed, surely in Italian, by the kinfolk she had left behind.

On Sunday, June 15, 2003, Silvia died at two in the afternoon. She was peaceful. Her lungs had filled with fluid. She breathed with difficulty, indeed, breathed the death rattle, but she was not in pain. So the hospice nurse told me.

John and I were on a desert mountaintop in a national forest in New Mexico outside Santa Fe. We received a call on my cell phone. At Silvia's request years before, John had made arrangements for her body to be donated to Washington University Medical School. Silvia wanted no formal funeral service, so John decided we should stay on in the West for a long-planned visit with Missy and Walt in Colorado. John slept little, was overactive and unreasonable. He argued with me that his mom had been dead for him long before our trip, argued with my sister and niece, wrote frantically on legal pads in the middle of the night. He screamed at me that he was not upset, not feeling guilty about hiking at the moment of his mother's death. By the time we returned home, I was exhausted, as if the weight of many years of death and dying had devoured me.

Our family and close friends gathered at our house late in June to celebrate Silvia's life.

Slowly, John and I began to swim to the surface.

—⁓—

At the end of June, Mom sent an e-mail. To her granddaughter Molly, Anna's sister. Her "teacher" at Villa Manor printed her cards to carry in her purse with her e-mail address and phone number. While Mom never used the computer after sending that initial message, she kept the cards in her purse for anyone who might ask. Maybe because of the shock of this high-tech world she had entered, Mom seemed very old when I took her out for lunch that afternoon. Her legs didn't want to swing into the car. Her knees couldn't hold steady when she stood up after lunch, so she plopped back down into her chair. It was hot and muggy; she was tired before we started our errands. At one point, she looked around the store: "No one else here has to use a walker."

"Okay, Mom, if you scan the store, you won't see any 91-year-olds in the aisles on this 95-degree day. Not in the Clinique aisle or by the Chanel perfumes."

She grumbled, "True, I don't see any. But I still don't understand why I need a walker."

"I don't hear you well, Mom," I said. Her voice was muffled. Rather than feeling comfortably entwined with her, I was impatient about this replay of the walker argument.

"I don't know," she opened her mouth wider and pronounced loudly, as if I were the old person, "why I need a walker."

As we drove home, she said, "You know, all my friends are off on adventures."

"The ones from the Friday reading group?"

"Off they go for the summer." She waved her hand as if they had vanished. "Betty's off in Maine—I don't see how she manages the trip. Lois drove herself to Colorado."

I knew not to intervene when Mom launched into an everybody-but-me-is-having-fun recitation.

"I could call Patricia, but she drinks two martinis at lunch. I don't like to ride with her. And Kate—she can't see a thing. I can't be in charge of her. I don't have any energy to organize."

"That leaves Maria, Mom." The Friday group was such an established part of Mom's life that I knew lots of details about the members and their foibles, even though I'd never been to one of the meetings.

"Oh, Maria. I can't understand her accent. And she has to bring that darling husband of hers because he can't be left alone. Of course, it's not bad to have a man around." She laughed at herself. In a low voice, she went on, "Do you know that I can't sing any more? Nothing comes out. Not even when I'm alone with Yummy. No hymns. No camp songs. No *Carmen*. None of that glorious music I used to know."

I could barely discern her words.

That muggy day, Mom was very much herself at 91 years old, the day she received and answered her first e-mail.

I felt guilty as I began to pack for Pentwater, guilty about leaving Mom, about resenting the space and energy she took in my life. George was in town and would look after her while we were away. Old people informed John's and my life on every front. A day or so before we left for Michigan, John went to St. Ambrose Church with a priest to sort out an 88-year-old client's possible divorce. The client had threatened to cut off funds from a family member. I was surprised that John, an avowed nonbeliever, would turn to a priest as a helpmate to reach this old guy. John, on the phone with the old fellow, sounded saintly. He was patient, willing to go over legal details, just as he had done with his parents. I wondered if these were lessons we had learned—be ever so patient; ask for help, even from unexpected sources; listen and then listen again. I did not want to embrace a life of constant, willing helpfulness. A perpetual caregiver of old, old parents, oh please, no, no.

Yet, I collided with the very old every day. On a sparkling July day that mirrored Michigan weather, as I walked with Rufus, I saw a woman who lived in an apartment building in our neighborhood. Well into her eighties, she always wore fantastic clothes. That day she wore gloves with fur cuffs, 1960s pink Bermuda shorts, a blue sweat shirt, and high heels with orange, rolled-down knee socks. She had no teeth at all, so her lips folded in on themselves. I pictured her daughter, maybe my age, living her workaday life far away and how she would gasp and roll her eyes if she could see her mother.

Daily, this flamboyant woman swept the sidewalks, gutter, steps, and walkway in front of her building.

On my walk, I happened onto that old woman's poetry.

I said, "You're out sweeping early today."

The old woman said, "I was just telling my father that we humans love this cool breeze."

"It is nice."

The old woman said, "But the trees hate the breeze. Look at all the twigs they've lost. The trees want water, not the breeze."

"Ummm."

"I'm here to clean up after the trees and their little twigs so that you'll be safe."

She chucked me under the chin affectionately. And if I were as lucky as she, on my walk I would talk to my own father. I yearned to talk with Dad again about the Silk Road and Kipling, to enjoy his stern, guarded manner and the blue of his eyes melting as he called me Chickadee. This must be what Pastor Daniel meant by holy ground.

I named the third week of July in Michigan the week of Dan Brown's novel, *The Da Vinci Code*. We remembered Pentwater summers by books: *Jaws* scared the children, but they couldn't put it down and didn't go into the lake for a few days for fear of sharks; *Jonathan Livingston Seagull* spawned earnest teenage discussions; I felt worldly and cynical when I laughed over *Bridget Jones's Diary*. The men read *Founding Brothers* in 2001. For several summers, *War and Peace* accompanied us but lay unopened by the chaise longue on the porch. In July 2001, John and I read *The Odyssey* aloud to each other. In 2003, it was the *The Da Vinci Code*. I read it first.

I staked out a claim to the wicker chaise longue and devoted myself to porch reading right after Will and Carol left for home with spouses and children. In an instant, I was transported to the grand gallery at the Louvre. My art history professor during junior year in Paris marched the class from David to Delacroix. He analyzed paintings of solemn classical oaths, grandiose battles, staggering horses in luminescent reds and blues. *The Da Vinci Code* returned me to Paris, to my own romantic year there. The pines, the sound of waves, the voices echoing from the dunes, John—they all faded as I read deeply into the book.

The telephone rang. I hopped up, finger stuck in the *Code* to mark the page. It was my mother in St. Louis, blessedly far away.

"Yes, beautiful weather, Mom."

"No, we're not busy. I'm not busy. Are you, Mom?"

"Well," she began "the other day, one of those poor lost souls who live here at Villa Manor stood up right in the middle of the dining room and said, 'I don't know my way back to my room.' What do you think of that?"

I automatically answered, though I knew from geriatric guides not to correct my mother, "You know, Mom, that woman has a disease."

Like a haughty heroine, Mom queried me skeptically: "What disease?"

I repeated, as I had so many times over the years: "Alzheimer's disease."

"You know, I don't believe in Alzheimer's disease." I heard her steely tone, as if it were a creed. Months before, when I had tried to talk about Paul and Silvia's illness or even Dad's, I knew Mom did not accept this destroyer disease. Instead, she denied and excised Alzheimer's from her belief system, as if it simply did not exist.

For a moment in Pentwater, as I luxuriated in reading to the sound of waves and afternoon breeze, I thought that I, too, might be able to leave behind old age and Alzheimer's disease. Just dismiss it as fiction like the books I was reading.

I wanted to know how this escape from the Louvre would play out. I fidgeted with my book. I was impatient with my mother's slow-paced, desperate denial of how some "old souls" evolved.

"Some kind person in the dining room showed her the way. But you know what happened?"

"No, Mom." My mind drifted to Brown's story line. Ah ha, so they broke through the bathroom window. But that false escape was a red herring. It was pitch dark in the Louvre Museum. I couldn't figure out how Langdon and Sophie would find their way down the emergency staircase as alarms began to sound and gendarme cars readied for the chase with the pan-pon of their sirens blaring.

Mom's voice came as a voice-over, "Well, when she got to the front desk, I was standing right there. She was confused all over again. So I pointed her down the way where the two corridors turn off. But she asked me, 'How will I know which way to turn?'"

"That makes me sad, Mom," I said, reconnecting with her. "Can you imagine what she must feel like?"

"Well, if you ask me, if there is an Alzheimer's disease, it can be pretty funny." She chuckled at the other end of the line.

Funny or frightening. Or heartbreaking. I looked out at the lake. Its steady afternoon waves broke white against the sandy shore. A neighbor in St. Louis swept the street as she communed with her father; another old woman lost herself in the halls of her final home. Dan Brown let his characters speed through Paris thwarting pursuers. Because his was just a story, they escape to safety.

—⁜—

Late in October one evening at bedtime, Mom fell in her bathroom, full of porcelain corners, a tiled floor, and YumYum's litter box. She couldn't get up, called out in a weak cry, scooted on her bottom to reach the pull cord that rang the nurses' station. Then ten days later, she fell again in the daytime. The "fall phone calls" I received from Villa Manor were prescribed by Missouri law. With each fall, came less steadiness and less activity. The circle contracted—diminished confidence, tentative balance, little activity, swollen feet, fright, another fall. Mom didn't hurt herself on the bathroom fall, just some bangs and bruises. As she told the doctor, "I didn't break anything."

The doctors and nurses agreed that there was no reason to investigate the cause of the falls because tests might subject her to discomfort. Today, medical wisdom has changed and would probably prescribe investigation of the falls. The two falls could have been caused by the side effects of a urinary tract infection, extra medications for that infection, tiredness from an outing away from her room, a glass of sherry with the Friday reading group, ill-fitting shoes, Yummy under foot, a minor stroke, or a heart incident. I was enough like my mother to wish we could know, then take action. These episodes highlighted how little control she had over her body. The falls awakened fears about her own dying. She thought cancer caused the urinary tract infections, just as she had equated a breast bruise with cancer; constipation resulted from colon cancer; a heart attack or stroke was predicted by the tingling in her fingers. She asked me, "How will I know when the moment of my death is upon me?"

I could not answer. I hoped the moment would be soft, with Yummy curled in her lap, hoped that she might be able to sing again. Maybe something from *Carmen* or a hymn, like "For All the Saints, who from their labors rest."

"You know," Mom said, "old people aren't meant to be such a burden to their children."

"I understand. You didn't plan it, Mom." I loved her enduring clarity.

"My campaign," she said, still the warrior, "would be to do something about all these burdensome, tiresome old people who sputter along all alone in places like this. That would be my campaign." Her voice was momentarily crisp, as if she had one more cause to organize. It faded. "I feel as if I'm a burden."

The truth was my parents and John's had dreaded the idea of being a financial burden. They had worked hard and saved amply for their old age. Because of each couple's accumulated funds, we were able to provide them with care far beyond the norm. John and I had the luxury of choices, of added private care like Sandra for his mother, of first-rate facilities that did not carry the stench of urine and dried feces and did not abandon the aged to the monotony of wheelchairs parked in front of blaring televisions for hours on end. For us, there was no specter of funds running out. In that, our parents had blessed us. All the legal documents enabling others to step in—powers of attorney and medical directives—were in order. And yet, neither couple had faced squarely the housing or caregiving needs of their old age, nor had they foreseen the emotional or psychological changes of their senior years. Perhaps they never imagined themselves so very ancient, in spite of their ancestors' remarkable longevity.

John and I vowed that we would improve upon our parents, swore that we would not—oh never, we had learned, we told ourselves—would not burden our children in any way whatsoever. We would adapt our housing at the appropriate moment, clean our messes of saved newspaper articles and recipes, prune our belongings, reform ourselves to avoid our parents' shortcomings, as we prepared for our late years on all fronts, foresaw problems, and devised prepackaged solutions. Oh yes, we would play the endgame more mindfully, more considerately in order to ease our children's middle years. John and I would not leave our offspring to improvise. That's what we had found ourselves doing every step of the way with our parents; we had invented our caregiving as we journeyed through four cases of Alzheimer's disease.

None of the four parents ever, I am certain, meant to weigh us down.

I felt a fierce burden especially on gray, November days.

Almost daily I had obligations to my mother: a call to the trust officer about a pharmacy bill, a chat with the charge nurse about her medications, conversation at a party with a friend who revealed Mom's mix-up over lunch dates, an errand or two for cat supplies or pharmacy items. I recognized the weight of caregiving when I chose calm, classical music rather than NPR news on the long drive home from a visit with her or when I crashed into a deep sleep in front of the TV at eight in the evening after time spent with Mom. But the burden felt heaviest at 4 a.m., when I often woke feeling sad about my mother. I wondered whether she, too, was having "a bad night" because of her arthritis and plantar fascia, neuropathy, and fear. Was she staring at the dark from under her quilt and asking if this were her dying night?

A Pilates class, tennis, coffee and outings with friends helped, as did a long ramble with John. He heard me out, reassured me, and generously offered a word of advice from the experiences he was trying to put behind him. With his new regimen of medications, he felt better. He was seizure-free. His eyes lit up as he said, "What would you think about a trip to Paris?" or "Let's get pizza tonight. You don't want to cook." With a jaunty step, he came alive. Waiters, once again, paused to ask if anyone had ever told him he looked like Spencer Tracy. He glowed.

Mom's voice grew weaker, her balance more tentative, her eyesight poorer. "Aren't those fountains over there?" she asked, as we glimpsed smoke stacks on a building. Perhaps they should be fountains, the Trevi Fountain or the Versailles extravaganza.

"Do you know that I can't sing any more?" she asked again. " I get out the hymnal and try to sing to Yummy. Nothing comes out."

"Yes, you've told me that, Mom."

Parts of her memory grew blurrier; her energy lessened; her verve turned from mauve to pale lavender. I mourned the graying of our parents' era, of my mother's life.

On November 26, I wrote the owner of the cottage in Pentwater. Please reserve three weeks for us in July of 2004. That would be, I reminded her, our thirty-third year in her cottage, my forty-fifth summer in Pentwater. Yes, I told her, John's health was now excellent; his combination of medications kept him on an even keel. He and I didn't know whether any of our children or grandchildren would be with us. We hoped, I wrote, that our daughter Carol would introduce our newest granddaughter, Anna Coleman, to Pentwater. But it was still too early for the children to plan, too many variables.

For me, the whole family would be there in Michigan: my mother and father, Paul and Silvia, my siblings, Nana Coleman and her brood of three children with their trunks arriving by train as they did in 1916. My parents would rent a cottage down the boardwalk. Ellen would shepherd Carol and Will as they prepared a family parade on the beach. Paul and Silvia would be ready for any kind of outing. Those sprawling bodies on the living room floor, heads covered by old blankets, were Ellen, Will, and Carol's college friends visiting for a weekend. Fireworks on the beach would celebrate family and the Fourth of July. Grandchildren Devon and Simon, twins Celia and Abby, and Sam would pad barefoot around the cottage, curling sand between their toes. My mother in her cottage would listen to *La Bohème* as she needlepointed a chair cover. With binoculars, my father would watch the lake for approaching storms. Paul would try to swim across the lake to Milwaukee in spite of the no-solo-swimming rule. Everyone would collect in Pentwater in July 2004. The first one awake in the morning would fetch sticky cinnamon buns and the day's papers from town. The most relaxed person would never move from the chaise longue on the porch. The last to climb the dunes from the beach at 6 p.m. would get cold water in the outdoor shower.

I would fall asleep as the wind quieted to a whisper in the pine trees, distant waves lapped the sand, and young voices downstairs played Scrabble in July.

12

The Egyptians
2004–2006

At the end of 2003, I told myself I'd had enough of keeping an "old people's book," as I called my journal. My mom—the last of our parents—and I relished each other's company more than ever before. Her spunk tickled me and made her timeless. So no more chronicling her decline. Ten years, basta, enough, no more, put the old people and their Alzheimer's disease behind you, enjoy life a little, pack some swimsuits and rain gear and go with John on his dream trip to Machu Picchu and the Galapagos Islands. A bit of our own bliss.

I decided, however, to use my old people's journal as the basis for this book.

I did not take notes at one of Mom's medical checkups when she complained about being bored. The doctor, a handsome rascal, who was Dad's and Mom's longtime internist, said to my mother, sitting in the wheelchair she used on outings:

"Dorothy, you should take a trip. Susan here will take you to Paris or at least New York City."

Out of respect, I did not roll my eyes at the doctor. No way, at that phase of my life, when I'd realized the need to pamper myself with massages and physical therapy at the slightest twinge and give myself grandbaby trips and dinners out with John, no way would I haul my mom any place except to doctors and to the mall restaurant where she loved the popovers with honey butter.

Nor did I transcribe the visit to that same dashing doctor when Mom talked about YumYum.

"Doctor, my daughter here won't do it. Refuses. But, you, I'd like you to write an order."

"An order for what, Dorothy?"

"I want YumYum to be euthanized when I die and buried with me, cuddled right on my chest where she sleeps. You can write an order."

"That's not part of my medical practice."

"The Egyptians did it," said Mom, as persuasive as I'd seen her in ages.

"I can't do that. In spite of the Egyptians. This is between you and your family."

Immediately afterward, I got in touch with Missy and George with a heads-up: "Mom's got this euthanizing YumYum notion on the brain. Just know that I'll have no part of it—zero, nada, niente—nothing to do with it. And the doctor says no, too. So please don't ask me for help with this scheme. Yummy has many years ahead of her."

I laughed: what an arena to stand up for myself. No, no, and again no. And it all had to do with a cat I didn't even like!

Why make note of Mom's daffiness? I dug into volunteer activities, grandmothering, transforming my old people's journal into a book, traveling coast-to-coast to visit family, and taking excursions far and near with John. To college reunions—we were both groupies who loved everything about college life—and to London, Paris, Venice, and Mexico, as if, parched after years of looking after our parents, we were at last drinking from a deep, bubbling spring.

My wry sense of humor crept back. John and I, my siblings and I, could, with a dark comedy streak, flesh out some of Mom's adventures, although I knew in the well of my being that these adventures signaled more than mere balminess.

In the fall of 2004, she and Betty T. decided to meet in a mall midway between their dwellings. They planned lunch, maybe a movie, a bit of shopping: two nonagenarians—one with a walker, one with a cane—converged by taxi. Each had a taxi charge card. At this time, both were still deemed "independent" by family and aides, including me. But as the afternoon drew to an end and dusk came, Mom and Betty needed to phone the cab company for two separate cabs. Neither had a cell phone. I imagined these two willful and mighty 90-somethings in consultation:

"Dottie, let's think: how will we call the taxi?"

"Betty, we need a phone booth."

"Dearie, phone booths don't exist any more. Have you seen one anywhere?"

"But there must be phones just around on the wall."

I imagined the two clumping down the mall's walkway, white-haired heads raised like turtles peering left to right to cross a road. Ah, a public phone.

"Betty, do you have the number of the cab company?"

"We have to use our heads, Dottie. Don't you imagine the number's on the charge card?"

"I might have some coins. I wonder how much it costs to make a call these days. Remember, Betty, when our phone numbers began with letters? I still remember PA for Parkview."

It was at about this moment that I'd received a call from the front desk of Villa Manor, where my mom had signed out at 11 a.m.

"Susan, do you have your mother with you?"

"No. Why?"

"Just wondering. She signed out and left in a cab several hours ago."

My mother's arthritic fingers and rheumy eyes could neither see coins in her black coin purse nor pick them up. Betty, meanwhile, fumbled, I imagine, among her credit cards and museum membership identifications for the taxi charge card with its phone number.

As Mom later told me, gleeful at being able to tweak me with her near-miss adventures, right then a saleswoman from a department store was leaving for the day. She came upon these two befuddled, once potent, women. She asked if she might help.

"The dear woman," my mom told me, "led us back into the store. She called for two taxis and told them where to meet us. We would never have known how to do that, Betty and I. And she took us to the door and waited with us. It all turned out so well."

After Mom's next taxi adventure, I had to weigh in, confiscate the charge card, and cancel the account. On a fall afternoon at about 5 p.m., I set out on a walk with Rufus—jeans, walking shoes, a springy step. At the intersection between our dead-end street and a major cross-town boulevard—about one block from our house—a taxi made a turn onto our street. It slowed as it proceeded, as if the driver were searching for a number. I happened to glance into the back seat as the taxi passed me. My mother, it was Mom riding up our street. Could it really have been Mom? I turned, dragged Rufus along, and ran after the taxi. I hailed the cabbie, who pulled over. There was Mom in full cocktail party regalia in the back seat, trying to direct the cabbie to our house.

"Aren't you ready for the party?" My mother looked me up and down, eyed Rufus, mustered her maternal disdain. "You don't look at all ready."

"And I see you're ready, Mom," I said, studying her silk dress, earrings, pearl necklace, Ginger Flower lipstick, and gloves.

The cabbie intervened: "She described your house. Gray brick. She said I could let her off there for the party."

Rufus and I followed the cab carrying my mother, her walker, and her party purse with taxi charge card to our house. She paid the driver with her card. I unloaded her from the cab into my car, put Rufus in the house, and drove her back to Villa Manor, where she signed herself in and went to dinner.

In the kitchen between sips of wine, John and I laughed over hilarious visions of Mom camped on our front steps in silk dress and pumps, waiting for John or me to come home for the party. I realized, too, that Mom's imaginings could easily carry her into untenable situations. Although she thought I was demonstrating my "usual tendency to exaggerate," I insisted that the world held some dangers for a nonagenarian on the loose with credit cards, cash, and only a vague notion of where she lived.

I took the taxi charge card out of her wallet and asked Villa Manor not to allow or facilitate cab trips. Because Betty and Mom together were capable of carrying out any number of fantastic outings, I consulted with Betty's son, who agreed to impose the same restrictions.

For several years, I never gave a name to what was happening to Mom, because for her, Alzheimer's disease was taking a flamboyant shape, an adventure format—very different from Paul's, Silvia's, and Dad's manifestations. Why had I not allowed myself to realize that Mom would walk offstage dramatically?

As for me, it was denial, yes, oh, that old muddy river de Nile. Or was it hard-learned self-preservation? I answered the 10 p.m. phone calls, once again resounding with the voice of the harried charge nurse: It's the charge nurse to let you know your mother's fallen on the floor in her room, on the bathroom tile, on the foyer rug tangled in her walker; no bruises, good spirits, just keeping you posted, good evening, yes, do have a good evening.

It occurred to me that I might keep a simpler record of Mom's decline, pencil in the dates of her falls on my day planner: February 25, 2006; February 27, 2006; March 19, 2006; April 18, 2006. I also marked: Mom, urinary tract infection. The next day, in between my Pilates class and the planting of a new bay magnolia tree, I wrote, in my shorthand, that Mom's psychiatric nurse practitioner had increased her dosage of antidepressant. On April 26, 2006, in the evening, Mom fell, kerplunk, trying to catch YumYum for what I supposed was a good-night cuddle. Two days later, she fell at her Friday reading group at Betty T's house. Another friend who'd been there phoned me in dismay. They had called the police because no one could lift her. Mom reported how embarrassed she was but how charming the police officer had been. He volunteered to help any time. I was wary, once again frightened at the course of events.

I was not surprised when first the charge nurse, then the administrator, telephoned to tell me that Mom needed more care, more surveillance. She would, they announced, have to move to the first-floor, skilled nursing unit, a locked unit with its own enclosed garden and dining room. A small unit, the hallways of patients' rooms ran diagonally, like spokes of a wheel, into a central nurses' station as the hub. As soon as a single room opened up (when someone died), Mom would move. Yummy was welcome to go with her.

Moving day was a bright, balmy day in May 2006. The nursing

home had helped plan logistics and assigned someone to lift and transport heavy furniture, like the tall writing desk. George, who certainly would have helped, was in Tuscany, where he always spent two months in spring and two in fall. And John had appointments with clients and meetings scheduled all day. I transferred Yummy first, so she would not be underfoot as I packed and wheeled boxes on a dolly to Mom's new room. I closed YumYum in Mom's new bathroom with familiar toys, one of Mom's blankets, the litter box, food, and water. While I knew this was not ideal for a cat, it was the best system I could devise. A nurse was assigned to Mom for the day. With that one-on-one attention and the promise that Yummy could stay with her, Mom took the move in stride.

After YumYum's move, I was stopped abruptly by Reba, the second-in-charge nurse's aide in Mom's new unit.

"You her daughter?" Reba jerked her head at Mom's new room.

"Yes, Dorothy's my mom." I was friendly, ingratiating. I'd learned from experience that we needed every single staff member on our team. I took time to schmooze, to chat about the staff members' children and vacation plans.

Reba tipped her head in a watch-out-for-me way: "I don't do cats. I'm not going into your mother's room. Ever. Cats aren't in my job description."

I set down the load of clothes I was carrying at the nurses' station. "Well, everyone loves YumYum." I was unprepared, focused on moving furniture and pictures, anxious about Mom's well-being as she adjusted to a narrower world in this unit.

"I'm going to see the supervisor. I tell you, I don't take care of cats. I'll give you the sheets to make her bed. I won't go in her room. Do you hear?" Reba's tone was aggressive and mean.

I reloaded my arms. Heavy-hearted, I mechanically rehung suits, summer print dresses, Saturday play clothes, and shirtwaists, as Mom called her many blouses—silk for suits, flowered short-sleeved for summer, oxford cloth or denim to wear for physical therapy. How to find a way to appease Reba, how? I needed to count on her support, for she was on duty most weekdays. I plodded through the move, head down as I passed the nurses' station, load after load. I stopped to hug Mom as she ate lunch in her new dining room.

I was almost finished with the move when I saw Reba again in the corridor. She bounced up to me:

"Your mother founded Planned Parenthood in St. Louis?"

"Not really. Why? She was just there early on. Why do you ask?"

With the same feisty tilt of her chin, Reba said, "That's her portrait in the Planned Parenthood headquarters, isn't it? I've seen it lots of times."

"That is my mom."

"The others here, they all know." She waved her arm towards the nurses' station. "Your mom's the Planned Parenthood lady. Miss Susan, can I do anything for your mother? I'm taking towels to her room right now. And I'll check on everything. On the cat, too."

13

Independence Day
2007

As part of my New Year's resolution to enliven Mom's existence, I invited myself to go with her to a reading group lunch at Betty T's home. She needed a driver and a companion, preferably a family member like George, Anna, Missy's daughter who was working in St. Louis, or me. Mom had grown confused, sometimes combative, but mostly disoriented and could no longer go out alone.

As the reading group members sipped sherry, Betty began, "Do you remember dancing at the Starlight Roof?" She bobbed her head at the circle of friends, my mother, and me.

"What? Where?" Patricia turned her good ear toward Betty.

"Patricia, we're talking about dancing at the Starlight Roof," repeated Kate, her white hair majestic in its curved bob. She wore sunglasses even in the watery January light, for she was legally blind, sighted enough to see a good deal but not to read or drive. "When I was growing up in Rhode Island, we went to the Arthur Murray studio to learn to dance."

"Oh my, remember those dancing lessons?" Patricia added. "I hid in the dressing room." She took a drink from her sherry. "But I did learn how to go through receiving lines."

"Nowadays, the young people don't even touch when they dance," said Lois. In her early eighties, the youngest of the group, she represented the voice of youth for the others.

Everyone laughed. Except Mom, who was a beat behind. She stared at each of her friends, as if for an explanation. They seemed to avoid her gaze as their chuckles faded.

"I was thinking of Chandler and how he could dance," said Betty, fingering the knot in her silk scarf. "Remember Chandler?" Betty pushed herself up to standing. With her cane, she crossed her living room to the grand piano where photos in silver frames stood in rows. She reached out a gnarled hand for one picture. "Here I am with Chandler."

"What a dancer he was. And so dashing," Patricia said. She wore a tweed suit, pumps, and nylon hose.

Mom appeared to watch her four oldest, dearest friends, who'd gathered for lunch on this Friday as they had done for decades. Even though they still called themselves the reading group, reading aloud was nearly impossible because of Patricia's and Betty's deafness, Mom's decline and detachment, and Kate's blindness. That left Lois to drive the group to the gathering spot, to choose articles, and to be the reader.

Betty passed the picture around the circle: Chandler, slim and dapper, wore a white suit with a long scarlet scarf. Betty was dressed in a patterned silk gown.

"A beautiful dress. Such a dancer. Didn't you love it?" each woman murmured, for a moment lost in a memory, I imagined, of the elegance and romance of the early 1930s.

"You know," Betty began, "if I didn't have all my S-T-U-F-F, we wouldn't have this picture of Chandler. It would all be cleared out." She waved her hand over her living room with its 12-foot-high ceilings: shelves of leather-bound books, master drawings in gilt frames, back issues of the *Journal of the United Nations* and *Foreign Affairs*, and that day's *New York Times*. The soft taupe carpeting, the fireplace burning orange with licks of blue flame, and the chintz-covered chairs invited guests to sit and stay awhile. "Emily came over and told me I needed to get rid of all my S-T-U-F-F. She always spells the word to make it seem worse."

"Who's Emily to say? She's just your daughter-in-law," said Lois.

"She retired in June. She thinks she should organize me," said Betty.

Kate said, "Well, we have to find something else for Emily to do. What are her interests?"

"All those years, she was a math teacher. But her degrees are in art history."

A buzz went around the room. The women brainstormed. They pooled their volunteer experience and connections until a consensus built.

"A docent at the art museum," the cry went up. "A teacher. Art. A natural. Besides, it has a two-year training program. She'll be busy. Perfect."

"I want my S-T-U-F-F around me. It's my whole life," said Betty. "Let's have lunch, girls, now that we've solved what to do with Emily."

The custom was that every woman brought her own sandwich and that the hostess furnished sherry, coffee, and dessert. Kate, Lois, and Patricia each arrived with a brown bag.

I retrieved my mother's walker. The security belt I used to hoist her up the outside steps lay with a box of Kleenex in the walker basket. Hands under her armpits, I lifted her to a standing position. Her swollen ankles wobbled. "I'm up," she said. The aluminum of the walker clattered as she wheeled into the dining room.

Betty's son had set the table on his daily morning visit: plates with exuberant purple pansies, lavender table linens, crystal water glasses—all on a shiny mahogany table. One by one, the women pulled out plastic bags and dropped sandwiches on their plates—two squares of thin white bread from which a curl of lettuce and the edge of a slice of processed turkey or ham dangled. I had transgressed by buying two giant sandwiches on crusty peasant bread, tomato and provolone cheese slices on a stack of smoked chicken with pesto. I abandoned one of our sandwiches in the kitchen and served Mom and myself a half sandwich each to be more in line with the other women's lunches. After all, this was my first time to attend the reading group.

"Dottie dear," Betty said, "aren't you lucky to have Susan along?"

"I'm so lucky to be here." My mother's shoulders seemed to relax with her first words of the day. "But I'm not sure I can get my mouth around this sandwich Susan bought me," she said in her familiar wry tone.

Her friends tut-tutted in agreement.

I watched, wondering if I needed to cut Mom's sandwich. I didn't want her to drop bits of her sandwich on herself or her placemat, not here with these beloved friends. But then I noticed for the first time that the mauve cotton jersey top and pants a nurse had chosen for her were already caked with food, probably from breakfast. Underneath, peeking above the V-neck of her top, she wore an angora cardigan. Why an outer sweater underneath? To ward off the January chills? From confusion about the order of clothes? Where was my impeccably groomed, well-dressed mother? She wrapped her hand like a claw around the sandwich and bit down. Crumbs showered down her front.

"Did you read the article in the paper about modernist houses? You know, the ones from the fifties," asked Kate.

"It's a pity, a shame." Patricia dabbed at her mouth with her napkin.

Lois announced, "I'm categorically opposed to tearing old buildings down."

"All those beautiful houses in the woods, so connected to the outdoors, like Nan and Henry's—I loved going there." Kate's sunglasses sat by her plate. Her large eyes looked watery.

"Girls," Betty said, "we have to do something to stop this. We can't let others tear down all the best architecture in town. What shall we do?"

"You're right, Betty dear."

"Letters to the editor. We need to write the paper. Who do we know?"

Voice overlapped voice; bread with turkey lay abandoned on plates; plans of action from these veterans flew around the table. Mom bent her head to her slab of sandwich. I watched—her disengagement from the conversation, the effort it took her to eat, the stains on her clothes, the mussed hair that neither the nurse nor I had remembered to comb. I was overcome by grief for my mother's decline yet exhilarated by the din of these ancient women.

"Betty dearie, what's that package at your place?" Lois changed directions.

"An early birthday present. A former student. He always thinks my birthday is in January."

"It's in February. You have another month until you're ninety-six," Patricia teased Betty.

"I love presents." Betty's nail tore at the wrapping. Kate offered to help. Lois noticed Kate's shiny rose nails. "Your polish is so perfect." The women admired each other's manicures, and I was pleased that Mom still had her nails done every week.

"It's a book. Oh, Calvin Trillin. I do love him," Betty said.

"Aren't you in luck? Read me the title, Betty," Kate said. "He's marvelous. I hope it's on tape."

"Who's Calvin Trillin?" my mother asked.

Patricia touched my mother's arm gently and said, "I'm sure you've read his pieces in the *New Yorker*, Dottie."

"Oh yes, oh yes." My mother drank her coffee.

"It's a love story. I heard about it on NPR. And look at how handsome they are," Lois said. "Let's pass it around."

"In fact," Betty passed the brownies after the book, "it could be our reading today. I'd love to hear a love story."

My mother shifted, squirmed in her place. Time had run out. She turned to me, "I'm tired. I need to go home right away." An inner clock, her bladder, the call of Yum Yum, I didn't know why this was the moment.

I found her walker, her old blue angora coat, and attached the security belt. Patricia held Mom's elbow as I grasped under one arm and gripped the belt with my other hand.

"Dottie, we love having you with us. We love it. So many years together, dear," Patricia guided Mom's legs as they swung into my car.

As we drove west on the highway, I asked Mom how she'd enjoyed the outing.

"It was thrilling," she said, "thrilling."

"I'm glad. You have wonderful, loyal friends."

"I found it," my mother paused, "stultifying."

"What do you mean?"

"Maybe that's not the right word." She pulled her coat tightly around her neck.

I kept my eyes on the afternoon traffic.

"I was sad," she said. "Everyone is so old."

—⁓—

In February, the charge nurse called me for a "discussion." Mom was stirring up other residents about the food, urging them not to eat.

Later that day, Mom phoned me: "I'm organizing a fund-raiser. I need a donation from you."

"What for, Mom?"

"For food."

"Food?"

"My friends and I are going on a strike to protest the terrible food here. I need to provide some alternative food. I need money."

The charge nurse had told me that my mother's agitation might necessitate an intervention—a visit from the psychiatric nurse or a calming medication. I thought of Mom's lifelong distaste for the type of "slap-dash" food served at Villa Manor: scoops of cottage cheese with hard, unripe melon; sloppy, unidentifiable meat on a tasteless white bun. I didn't dare tell the nurse how cheered I felt that Mom was willing to raise her voice. If the Villa Manor staff had bothered to read my mother's biography, summarized in her admissions papers, they might have interpreted the former activist's behavior as a sign of improved mental health.

No interventions were needed. The food strike never materialized because no one agreed to supply the rebels with alternative food, and Mom didn't have a backup plan.

—␣␣—

At my annual physical exam, my doctor, who had spiked red hair, wore capri pants and high-heeled mules showing her painted toenails, suggested, apropos of nothing, that I try meditation, that it would be a good life skill for me to develop. I wondered, as I drove home, what had led her to that suggestion? My blood pressure, reflexes, lungs, and ears were normal. I'd mentioned, rather breezily, that I was involved in elder care for my mother. I promised myself I'd replay the entire examination in my mind as soon I got home to see what I had revealed that prompted the meditation suggestion. One quick glance in the rearview mirror showed me the image the doctor had perceived: a face drawn in shades of more than a decade of grief, sadness, devotion, anxiety, love, and anger. A face I'd taken for granted, left unnoticed for years. Perhaps, rather than praying for help, I would meditate.

—∞—

As recommended by Villa Manor, Missy, George, and I engaged hospice care for our mother beginning on Easter weekend 2007. I'd taken Mom to her reading group three months ago, and only two months had passed since the planned food strike. Now, our mother was immobile, incontinent; she rarely spoke and jumbled her words when she tried. She seldom opened her eyes, ate on occasion, but at this point she was scarcely the mother any of the three of us had known. There would be palliative care, even time with a hospice music therapist; Mom would be comfortable.

One hospice aide, a good-looking young man whom I'd met several times, had wheeled Mom on a stroll through Villa Manor. He always phoned me after each of his visits with Mom.

"I wheeled your mom around to all the first floor rooms. I couldn't tell if she even had her eyes open or was listening to my chat. I carried on about the activity room with its birds in cages and the wicker room with its watercolor show. Not a word from her. We got to the club room. You know, the dark room with leather chairs and the little bar where they hold Friday Happy Hour?"

"I do," I answered. "I know the room."

"So I said to your mom, 'Dorothy, do you recognize this room?' as I wheeled her in."

He went on: "For a second, she lifted her head. I stepped in front of the wheel chair to talk to her. She said, clear as day, her blue eyes on me:

'I'll have a bourbon on the rocks.' Then she dropped her chin and seemed to fall back into her halfway world."

"That was vintage Mom, sharp and ironic, funny as could be. I'm so glad you had a glimpse of her that way," I said.

With her Siamese cat, Yummy, as constant companion, Mom seemed to be living in a halfway world between her earlier life—with party frocks in swirling silk patterns and the promise of a cocktail in the evening, her life with causes to defend and family to counsel, the life she had lived fully and was now barely living—and a life to come on some other side. She had perchance already entered a new reality behind her closed eyelids and dipped chin. I wondered whether her ears heard music from that other side—music my father, her brother and sister, and parents all heard in their domain, where they were never alone or swimming solo but always together, listening to the cigarette song from *Carmen* or a hymn for all the saints or a tune about an enchanted evening.

At the end of June 2007, I baked chocolate chip cookies to take to my mom. Like Dad, her taste for chocolate never abandoned her. It was a warm Saturday afternoon. Mom was in her wheelchair, sitting under an umbrella in the nursing home garden with Cleo, the charge nurse.

"Cleo," she was saying, "you ought to consider more schooling."

"Hi Mom. I've brought some cookies."

"I'm busy interviewing Cleo for a more advanced job. But I will have a cookie."

"Not for me, thanks," Cleo said.

"Now, as I was saying, you have to set your sights higher than this, Cleo." My mom swept her arm across the garden and the doors back into the nursing home. "You're a woman of considerable gifts."

"Mom," I said, "you're in great shape today."

She turned in her wheelchair and fixed me with her blue eyes as if I were a stranger, "And what, may I ask, do you do in life?"

"I'm your daughter Susan, Mom. I've just dropped by to give you some cookies."

I was awestruck by my mom's "interview" of Cleo, by her unexpected acuity. I couldn't help, however, gulping hard when she asked what I did. Didn't she know me? Did she not understand that being there for her was what I was doing? When my brother visited her, Mom scrambled him with the many Georges who had peopled her life: her brother George, her husband George, the Episcopalian priest George. On the phone, my brother and I tried to laugh off Mom's muddle of our identities. Yet, memories of Silvia's queries about who John was and of Luciana's despair when her mother didn't recognize her haunted me. When Silvia mistook John for one of his uncles, he began to grieve for his lost mother. I was on the same trajectory.

I knew without asking that the end was near when, a few days after Mom's amazing interview with her, the unit administrator told me to find a new home for YumYum within a week. Mom's door needed to stand open. Hurrying nurses could not risk falling over a cat. The kitty litter box and bag of cat chow would have to give way to medical gear and supplies. YumYum went to live with a Villa Manor nurse whose son longed for a pet.

From her bed, Mom mumbled: "Yummy's gone, isn't she?"

"Yes." My voice caught. "Mom, your door has to stay open, so Yummy couldn't be safe here. She's in a good home with a little boy who'll give her lots of love."

Yummy was gone, and so was my mother. I asked myself what I would do with the rest of my life after all these caregiving years.

Dorothy died on Independence Day, 2007. She was 95 years old. A fierce thunderstorm broke over the cemetery just after her body was lowered into the ground. Missy, George, all of our children, and I gathered in a group hug, like a rugby scrum, and burst into singing. First, our old camp song, "To Northway Lodge we will return," then "O God, our help in ages past, our hope for years to come." John, Walt, Gabriele, and the pastor waited patiently as we hugged in a family knot.

I celebrated my mother in Pentwater two days after her funeral. I thanked her for the gift of July with deep family bonds and customs wrought long ago—no solo swimming, family sticks together, evening gatherings begin at 6 p.m., let's have a parade on the beach. I praised her for summers where Lake Michigan's waves and pine forests grant me a peace beyond all understanding.

Afterword

Fourteen years had passed between the summer day when Paul first swam solo straight out into Lake Michigan and the day of Mom's death. John, our family, and my circle of friends were my buoys against despair and solitude during those fourteen years of navigating dark, caregiving waters. When I faded, someone shone a beacon from a lighthouse. In times when John and I struggled, unanchored and without apparent aids, the people around us tossed us lifelines. John and I learned that we were not swimming alone.

I learned, too, that the very parents who had pulled us unwittingly into these deep waters of dementia never stopped being their beloved selves. The fearsome disease temporarily tainted but did not obliterate my appreciation of any one of them. When disease transformed them, they became different, sometimes insulting and accusatory. Alzheimer's disease stripped away their dignity. John and I attempted to convince ourselves not to take their words or utter confusion personally. Not that my heart did not drop into my shoes when Dad repeatedly called me a fraud; not that John's heart did not break when his mother showed no sign of recognizing him. Beyond that disease, beyond it lay what our parents harbored of their true selves, often invisible and inaccessible in the vortex of dementia. We tried to give them time and opportunities for their personalities to continue to show through. Paul, purposeful, charming and Venetian to the core, met people and exchanged greetings with his accustomed bonhomie until the end. My father, George, commanding yet tender, ate chocolate and saluted his nursing home public on his 91st birthday, four days before his death. Silvia—our dear, resilient, warm, practical Silvia—cared for her plants and then vanished for most of her final year. My mother, Dorothy, interviewed an employee, had her hair done, and ordered a cocktail—all in her last month.

Regrets: Do John and I have regrets about our efforts? We still walk Rufus, rain or shine, plunged in conversation about how we could have done more. Medically and financially, we think we managed well enough. We jump a puddle, skirt ice on the sidewalk, tug on Rufus's leash to keep him moving, for he is old, as we have grown older, too. While we walk, we mull over the final quality of life, especially for our mothers, who lingered long. John and I ran out of quality-of-life energy and imagination before our parents ran out of life. I should have culled the abundant materials about Alzheimer's and dementia we had collected to find better coping strategies with all four parents. I wish I had kept music playing for my mom; I wish I had read aloud to her, brushed her hair, massaged her gnarled hands. John wishes he had leafed through photo albums with his mother, even when she appeared to nod off. We could, at least, have asked the nursing staff to enhance the last months or years. We didn't. We were too tired, too ready after all the struggles for our mothers' lives to end.

I taught my students the French "r" from Edith Piaf's song, "Je Ne Regrette Rien" ("I Regret Nothing"). Though my French "r" rolls well, I do have regrets.

Looking back, I am unlike Piaf for I have regrets. Going forward, I must, like Piaf—a waif up from the streets of Paris, boldly singing her way into the hearts of French people—forge ahead in the next decades of my life. John and I walk and talk about this, about living forward without fear. Yes, we both know that Alzheimer's disease felled our parents. John has heard of other possible examples of the disease among family in Italy. Venetian relatives have recounted John's paternal grandfather's senility at the end of his life in the 1950s. But who in the medical community knows the degree to which Alzheimer's disease is inherited? Who can name all the factors that surely activate it, as well as any certain steps to keep it at bay? With genetic testing a possibility, how would either of us deal with the results, especially if they were positive?

So we walk Rufus, even with snow on the ground, on the uneven, 100-year-old sidewalks of our neighborhood. We grumble to one another about the hazards of winter walking. We need the companionship of quiet, uninterrupted chat, our connection to the seasons, the day's weather, the holiday decorations, the casual greetings that link us to our community. We are admittedly wary of the steps ahead, but neither he nor I will stay indoors out of fear.

Don't get me wrong. Fear hovers when I forget my glasses, cannot recall a friend's name, or when John overlooks two appointments in a row. Fear seizes at my throat, silences me—temporarily. But I remind myself that my father grew confused in his 89th year, when he phoned me in Pentwater over and over again about his auto insurance. He died just after his 91st birthday. That means he was compos mentis nearly 98 percent of his days. My mother began her theatrical exit—taxiing to our house for a cocktail party she imagined; her "food strike" at Villa Manor—at about 93. Except for the months of 2007 before her death, she remained great company.

Paul and Silvia had a bumpier ride. For the first few years of Paul's decline, we were clueless about what was happening. Neither John nor I knew a thing about Alzheimer's disease. To us, Paul's lost keys and cranky demands seemed merely the signs of old age. However, his behaviors were exaggerated—clinical symptoms of the disease, as we later learned. When Paul called from Madrid to ask John to send his forgotten hearing aids via diplomatic pouch, we thought this was eccentricity. Paul did have several rough years. Silvia endured the longest, most desperate years of dementia. Yet, nearly 85 of her 91 years were devoted to family, gardening, and welcoming guests.

Out of fear, John and I carry a flashlight when we walk after dark in the winter. Its beam lights only a small circle in front of us. Beyond the white circle lie unseen cracks and dark tree roots to traverse before we come home.

Regrets, yes. With Piaf's greatest song, we ponder the immense "If": "If the sea should suddenly run dry. . . ." Piaf's words ring in our ears, through the winter nights, through our fear. On our walks together, I have learned the power of love and loyalty from John, who, in the midst of his own problems, never flagged.

I move onward with an enduring sense of place, our family's special Pentwater. That tiny village enfolds all of us, where every year a family parade marches through our memories at sunset across the sand, as the hum of Dad's chant floats over the calm evening waters of Lake Michigan. The water, the mossy stairs from the beach through pine and birch forest to the old rust-red cottage inhabit my soul. Our three children, grandchildren, parents, my sister and brother, in-laws and their children, and ancestors all dwell in the slamming screen door, in the creaky metal bed frames, in the permanently damp Scrabble board, in the lumpy queen's chaise longue, in the little red bedroom reserved for the youngest child, in the dented aluminum kitchen pots, and in the out-of-tune piano. In that cottage, I can sing hymns of praise to the God who led me north to our place atop a sand dune in the midst of green woods, looking over a lake that shades from turquoise to azure to the dark blue of its deepest, coldest water. Here, I savor the joys of living distilled in the month of July. Here, too, I can play with a plunk, plunk on those chipped ivory piano keys, a song in a minor key for the profound and sacred darkness I shared in the aging and dying of the four old people whose lives and departures are chronicled in *Swimming Solo*.

Here is, then, my story of learning, through lake swims and beach parades, through disease with its folly, through loving and stress-laden moments, through neighborhood walks. This is my story of a family sticking together, ever reminded that no one, not a one of us, swims alone, rule or no rule.

July will find us walking the beach again in Pentwater, sand between our toes, waves splashing our ankles, intent on conversation or silent in our companionship. Our eyes will lift to the horizon, the far and vast horizon of our cherished family.

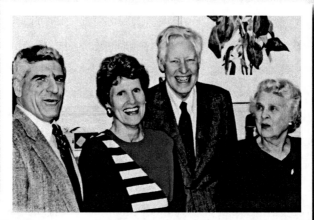

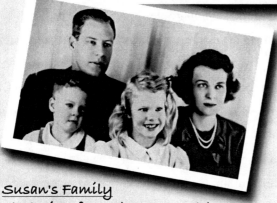

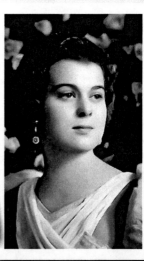

Susan's Family

Clockwise, from above: a World War II-era family portrait (George Jr. and Susan in front); John, Susan, George, and Dorothy at George's 85th birthday party; George as a young man; Dorothy in her 20s; Dorothy and George in the mountains

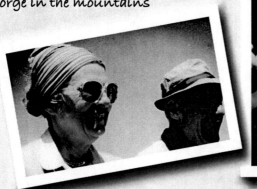

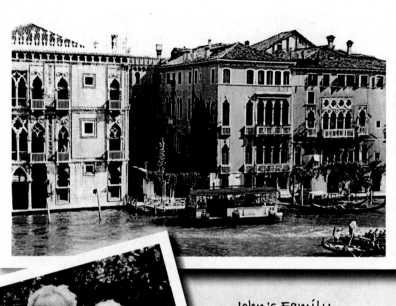

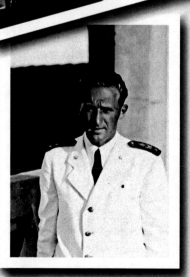

John's Family
Clockwise, from above:
Paul's family palazzo
in Venice, Silvia as a
young woman, Paul
in his Italian military
uniform, and the last
photo of Paul and Silvia

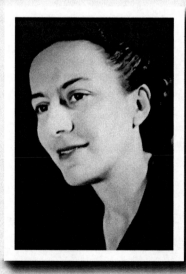

Acknowledgments

My thanks go out to the many people who have made *Swimming Solo* possible. I am, above all, grateful to our families. To John's siblings and mine, heartfelt gratitude for times shared, decisions forged, and extraordinary devotion to our four parents. A special thank you to my sister, Missy, for tennis therapy; to my brother, George, for a meticulous editorial reading; and to my sister-in-law, Luciana, for help on Italian facts and tales.

While at first the "old people's journal" that I kept was a coping mechanism recommended by a social worker, the entries grew into an outlet for my grief and astonishment at the changes in our lives because of Alzheimer's disease. In those first stages of writing, I never considered the possibility that a book would emerge.

As time and distance increased, my outlook changed. I realized that Alzheimer's disease begs to be explored and studied in hopes of deferring, deflecting, and, perhaps someday, curing it. I quickly learned that the disease alters and transforms caregivers as well as victims. I began to picture *Swimming Solo* as an offering, a teaching tool that might bring solace to other caregivers who feel alone and at sea in the midst of a dear person's dementia. I hope that this book demystifies the vagaries—unseemly and unexpected—of this dread illness, for then the tale of our parents' living and dying and our evolution as witnesses and participants will pay homage to the foursome.

My parents—George and Dorothy—and John's—Paul and Silvia—lived lives so full and so long that their stories are worth telling. Their vivid, sometimes bizarre declines highlighted their life adventures. I think of their gifts and legacies every day. Each parent had a bit of the teacher: my father, George, taught me Psalm 23 as my brother and I acted it out. My father came from teachers and preachers. My mother, Dorothy, taught high school English and mentored untold numbers of women committed to her causes. Paul, my father-in-law, began his career teaching law at the University of Padua in Italy. With her devoted, quiet manner, my mother-in-law, Silvia, taught my children to cultivate the garden and to prepare basil pesto.

Swimming Solo represents but one perspective, one set of family memories. From my point of view, our parents' stories offer lessons about cherishing life and plunging into it; about embracing family and civic responsibility; and about speaking up for tolerance, equal rights, and those who can't speak for themselves. In our parents' spirit, *Swimming Solo* tells their tales without hiding their accomplishments or shying away from the diminishment of Alzheimer's disease. To the four be the glory for great things they have done—and taught.

Thanks flow to my friends and fellow writers. Shannon Ravenel first edited and instructed me when I began to write about thirty years ago. Over many years, she has offered sage advice. The eight friends of our Talking Diners group—Karen and Steve Coburn, Peggy Guest and Frank Hamsher, Linda and Steve Skrainka, Madge and Tom Treeger—read an early version of the manuscript and contributed invaluable help and encouragement. Harriet Stone also read it with her insightful eye. I appreciate early readings from Bettye Dew and Constance O'Connor. Catherine Rankovic taught me in a creative nonfiction writers' workshop at Washington University and followed my manuscript through several stages. Caroline Kraus offered thoughtful advice about recounting family stories. The Three Rivers Writers Group helped, as several events set in Venice took shape some years ago. Finally, the Wild with Words writing group at Trinity Presbyterian Church gave me my first public reading.

This book would not have been possible without a bit of good luck. On a plane trip, I tore an article from the *New York Times* about a new publishing house. I followed with an e-mail, which led me to my publisher, Plateau Books, owned by Henry and Kathy Hamman. Henry is the acquisitions editor/business manager, and Kathy is the editor. Henry and Kathy have been unflinching in their support and perceptive commentary. The three of us have made quite a team. I am also grateful to Geoffrey Gerber, my lawyer, for his guidance through legal documents and to Jeff Hirsch for technical support.

Innumerable caregiving professionals made our roles easier. The Alzheimer's Association of St. Louis; J. William Campbell, M.D.; Consuelo Wilkins, M.D.; Pat Abernathy; Sharon Barnhart; Sandra Buchanan; Michelle Roberts; the two hospices that helped us and our mothers; and many others served our families as true care providers.

I save my warmest thanks for our immediate family—our children, Ellen, Will, and Carol—who, in their own ways, put up with a writing mom. Their love for their grandparents infuses this story, preserving good and poignant times. And, of course, all thanks to Gianni, my beloved partner, John, with whom I have sailed these waters, never alone. He has embraced my project, listened to iteration after iteration, and spoken up with editorial suggestions, fresh Italian family anecdotes, and acceptance of my focus on finishing *Swimming Solo*. Gianni, this book is for you—as a tribute and a love token, as a promise of more free time and open roads ahead.

St. Louis, June 2010

Resources

Organizations

AARP
601 E St., N.W.
Washington, DC 20049
888-687-2277
www.aarp.org

Alzheimer's Association National Headquarters
225 N. Michigan Ave.
Chicago, IL 60601
800-272-3900
www.alz.org
24/7 multilingual helpline: 800-980-9080 or 800-272-3900
e-mail address for sending questions: info@alz.org

Alzheimer's Disease Education and Referral Center (ADEAR)
P.O. Box 8250
Silver Spring, MD 20907
800-438-4380
www.alzheimers.org/adear

Alzheimer's Disease Research Center
Memory & Aging Project (clinical research office of ADRC)
4488 Forest Park, Suite 130
Washington University School of Medicine
St. Louis, MO 63108
www.alzheimer.wustl.edu

Centers for Medicare and Medicaid Services
7500 Security Blvd.
Baltimore, MD 21244
410-786-3000
www.cms.hhs.gov

Eldercare Locator
1112 16th St., N.W.
Suite 100
Washington, DC
800-677-1116
www.eldercare.gov

Family Caregiver Alliance
180 Montgomery St.
Suite 1100
San Francisco, CA 94104
800-445-8106
www.caregiver.org

Hospice Foundation of America
2001 S St., N.W.
Suite 300
Washington, DC 20009
800-854-3402
www.hospicefoundation.org

National Council on Aging
300 D St., S.W.
Suite 801
Washington, DC 20024
800-424-9046
www.ncoa.org

National Family Caregivers Association
10400 Connecticut Ave.
Suite 500
Kensington, MD 20895
800-896-3650
www.thefamilycaregiver.org

National Hospice and Palliative Care Organization
1731 King St.
Alexandria, VA 22314
800-646-6460
www.nhpco.org
www.caringinfo.org
Helpline, M–F, 9 a.m.–5 p.m. (EST): 800-658-8898

St. Andrew's Resources for Seniors
(Services in Missouri and Illinois; nationwide consulting and online resources)
6633 Delmar Blvd.
St. Louis, MO 63130
314-726-0111
www.standrews1.com

Books

Mace, Nancy L., and Peter V. Rabins. *The 36-Hour Day: A Family Guide to Caring for People with Alzheimer Disease, Other Dementias, and Memory Loss in Later Life*. (4th ed.). Baltimore: The Johns Hopkins University Press, 2006.

An indispensable, everyday guidebook.

Mittelman, Mary S., and Cynthia Epstein. *The Alzheimer's Health Care Handbook*. New York: Marlowe and Company, 2002.

A practical guide to caregiving with clear organization and key points. Useful information and strategies about hospitalization and end-of-life decisions, for example. Helpful appendices.

Petersen, Ronald, Ed. *Mayo Clinic on Alzheimer's Disease*. Rochester, MN: Mayo Clinic, 2002.

A readable work with large print, many illustrations, charts, and summary boxes. Four accessible sections with practical points. The "Quick Guides" for caregivers are especially useful.

Smith, Patricia B., Mary Mitchell Kenan, and Mark Edwin Kunik. *Alzheimer's for Dummies*. Hoboken, NJ: Wiley Publishing, Inc., 2004.

Trafford, Abigail. *My Time: Making the Most of the Rest of Your Life*. New York: Basic Books, 2004.

The author postulates a two- or three-decade bubble for people who have retired, an era of expansion, "generativity," contribution, and fulfillment.

Turkington, Carol, and James E. Galvin. *The Encyclopedia of Alzheimer's Disease*. New York: Facts on File, 2003.

A detailed source book with alphabetical references, many of which are scientific. About one-third of the book is devoted to resources, including organizations, sample documents, a layperson's bibliography, and a scientific bibliography. Excellent cross-referencing.

Discussion Guide

1. **Alzheimer's Disease:** As Susan Rava shows in *Swimming Solo*, each of the four parents exhibits his or her own particular Alzheimer's symptoms: Paul wanders; George is convinced his house and some mysterious family silver have been taken from him; Silvia loses most language; and Dorothy tries to organize a food strike, a cocktail party, and a job interview. Are you familiar with these characteristics? What symptoms have you had to deal with? How have you approached your loved one who may be afflicted with Alzheimer's? What suggestions can you glean from this memoir about dealing with Alzheimer's patients or those with dementia?

2. **Caregivers' Roles:** Throughout *Swimming Solo*, John, Susan, and others play evolving roles as caregivers. Compare scenes where their caregiver roles are the primary topic: John in chapters 3 and 4; Susan in chapters 7 and 11, for example. How did you react to Susan's honesty about her occasional negative feelings toward the parents? Have you been a caregiver? If you had been Susan, how would you have dealt with negative or anxious feelings? In what ways can you identify with the

caregiving roles and accompanying feelings in *Swimming Solo*? How are your experiences different?

3. Family Relationships: *Swimming Solo* tells the story of a family in crisis as it faces four cases of Alzheimer's. How does the family hold together during the years of caregiving? What role do George's beach parades play? Or Sunday lunches at Paul and Silvia's, later at John and Susan's? How do these events resemble your family's relationships? How does your family preserve its ties?

4. Caregivers' Stresses: John, Susan, their mothers, and other family members suffer from caregiver stress: anxiety, lack of sleep, crankiness, irrationality, distress, guilt, financial worries, and more. Experiences within the book differ: Silvia and Dorothy live round-the-clock with their spouses as the disease worsens. Several of John's and Susan's siblings live out of town at least part-time during the period covered in the book. Which family members—those near parents in St. Louis or those sometimes or always out of town—do you identify with? How might stresses for the two groups differ? Can you identify with the symptoms of stress illustrated in the book (for example, John's outbursts of anger; Susan's despair with her pastor; everyone's fatigue)? How have you coped with such stresses? What sources of help and relief have you discovered? What useful examples of coping did you find in Susan Rava's memoir?

5. Decision Making: After thought and consultation with family and professionals, John and Susan made what they thought were appropriate decisions about nursing home and assisted living placements, finances, and medical care. Caregivers in other families might choose different paths. John's and Susan's siblings might have made different decisions. Several scenes in *Swimming Solo* show different methods of family decision making. Compare John's family meeting with a social worker/care manager with Susan's lunch meeting with her mother. Given the information in *Swimming Solo*, what decisions would you have made differently, sooner, or later? What similarities and differences do you find between your family's decision making and decisions made in the book?

6. Institutional Placement: The decision to place a family member in an institution is one of the most difficult. All four parents in this book eventually live in institutions. The placements of Paul and George are vividly described. Has your family faced such placements? If so, how did you carry out the move? How did the family member placed in an institution react? Compare and contrast the similarities and differences between your experiences and those of individuals in this memoir.

7. Hospice, Death, and Burial: Susan Rava recounts the decision to engage hospice care for her mother and her mother-in-law. Hospice eased the circumstances of death for the two women. Paul and George both died suddenly without the need for hospice. Have you had experience with family members or friends in hospice care? If so, what kinds of experience? The funerals and burials of both fathers reveal more about the two men, celebrate some of their important traits, and recall the role of family ties. What parallels do you find with deaths and burials in your own family?

 8. Overview: Share any insights into yourself or others that you gained from reading *Swimming Solo*. In its exploration of family crises and Alzheimer's, how does this memoir succeed in celebrating the enduring qualities of family bonds?

9 780981 479507